# total
# meditation

# total
# meditation

susannah marriott

THUNDER BAY
P·R·E·S·S

San Diego, California

Dedication:
In memory of Haroon and Sophie

Acknowledgments:
Thanks to my yoga teachers, Rima and Nita Patel, and to the Sahaja yoga people for being in the right place (Broadstairs) at the right time (the folk festival). Thanks to everyone at MQP, especially Ljiljana and Leanne.

**Thunder Bay Press**
An imprint of the Advantage Publishers Group
5880 Oberlin Drive, San Diego, CA 92121-4794
www.thunderbaybooks.com

THUNDER BAY
P · R · E · S · S

Copyright © MQ Publications, 2004
Text copyright © Susannah Marriott, 2004

EDITOR Leanne Bryan, *MQ Publications*
EDITORIAL DIRECTOR Ljiljana Baird, *MQ Publications*
PHOTOGRAPHY Stuart Boreham
DESIGN Balley Design Associates
ILLUSTRATION Oxford Designers and Illustrators

ISBN 1-59223-196-9
Library of Congress Cataloging-in-Publication Data available upon request.

Printed in China

1 2 3 4 5 08 07 06 05 04

# introduction to meditation

Meditation has the potential to make a person happy. When scientists at the University of Wisconsin scanned the brains of practicing Buddhists, they discovered that the part of the brain associated with happiness showed much more activity than that in a control group of people who didn't practice meditation on a regular basis.

Meditation makes you happy in your body by enabling you to relax fully and release stress with muscle relaxation and breath control techniques. Meditation eases tension in the mind, too, by taking your focus away from worries and preoccupations. Meditation teaches you effective ways to deal with difficult emotions, such as anger and selfishness, and promotes techniques that develop compassion and love. Above all, meditation allows you to watch yourself and witness your life evolving. Armed with this self-knowledge, you start to change the way you behave for the better.

People who are happy spread happiness. When you approach work, relationships, and dealings with other people in an optimistic frame of mind, others respond to you in a more positive way. This deflates conflict before it arises and creates space in which to resolve problems. And the niceness builds: everybody you interact with gets a blast of your positivity and takes a piece of it with them into their own relationships. Meditation is a gift not just for you, but for your family, friends, coworkers, neighbors, and everyone else you interact with each day, from mail carriers to schoolteachers.

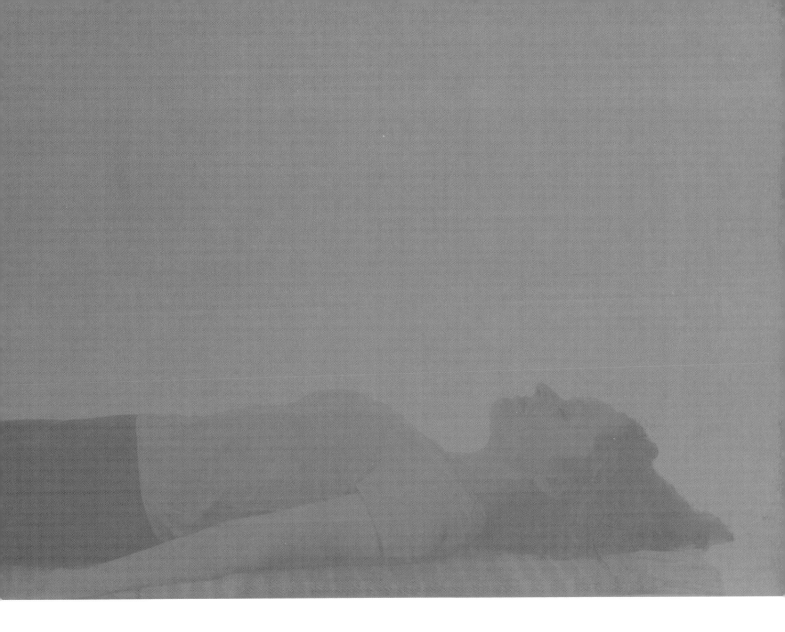

Happiness brings with it good health; people who consider themselves happy have been shown to have one-tenth the rate of serious illness and untimely death compared to those who consider themselves unhappy.

Meditation takes many forms, even though each path leads to a similar end. All the world's great spiritual traditions have developed methods over the millennia; medical science and sports psychology offer still more techniques. And then there is yoga, qi gong, and tai chi—all forms of meditation in motion. *Total Meditation* offers practical, easy-to-follow meditations from every tradition for the complete beginner. Whatever your reason for starting meditation, you will find something to suit you: relaxation techniques to release physical stress, nature walks to put you in touch with the environment, mantras, prayers, and puzzles to free your mind. There are methods for every time of day and night and for the office, car trips, and sports. Mindful music and sensory and breath techniques sit alongside conscious cooking, detox showers, and clearing clutter to simplify your life. Above all, there is the essence of meditation: just sitting in silence. I hope through these ideas you will find a way to be happy, just being and enjoying what you have right here, right now.

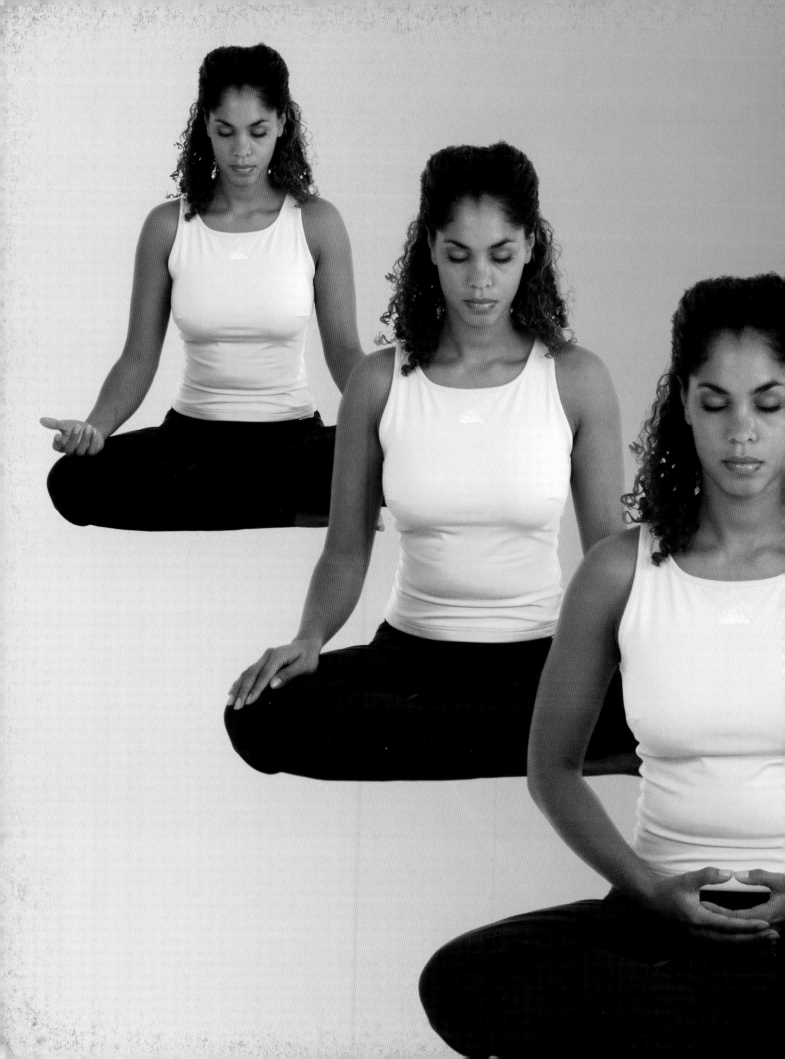

# why meditate?

# what can meditation do for me?

Many people approach meditation as another technique to study at an evening class, like aerobics or pottery; something that takes up an hour or so and is confined to a set time and place. But after a few sessions, people often realize that although meditation is this, it offers so much more. With practice, meditation becomes a mode of living and a new way of seeing everything: relationships, work, and home life; your future and your past. Along the way it can bring profound relaxation, increased mental clarity, inner peace, and spiritual enlightenment.

## what is meditation?

Meditation is simply consciously directing your attention in order to transcend the never-ending flow of thoughts through your mind. You can do it sitting still and silent with your eyes closed; you can do it by watching a candle flame, walking, practicing yoga, or studying a complex geometrical image; or you can do it by paying attention as you walk, cook, or clean, letting mindful activity block out other thoughts.

## find out about yourself

Meditation helps you discover more about yourself. When you imagine your mind as a wide screen and watch the incessant play of thoughts, sensations, and emotions that pan across it, you begin to realize that your thoughts, your anger or frustration, your aching leg don't define the "you" at your core. As you practice, you see that there is something inside that is more than these ever-mutating fancies. Using this self-knowledge, you gain understanding and insight. Your perspective widens and you reassess what is important and what isn't. Miraculously, answers to problems at home and work start to materialize.

## escape from yourself

When you meditate, you move inside yourself; at the same time, you step outside yourself. Being able to meditate helps you escape from the stranglehold of the ego, with its continual and overwhelming onslaught of desires, cravings, and demands. Freed from preoccupation with your interior state, you stop perceiving from your own perspective, where everything is colored with selfish thoughts, judgments, and comparisons, and with feelings of guilt and jealousy. You start inhabiting a new state of openness, ready to experience life as it comes. This is empowering and works well with the sense of self-determination that comes from knowing what your priorities are and believing you have the ability to work toward them.

"From meditation springs wisdom."

**The Buddha**

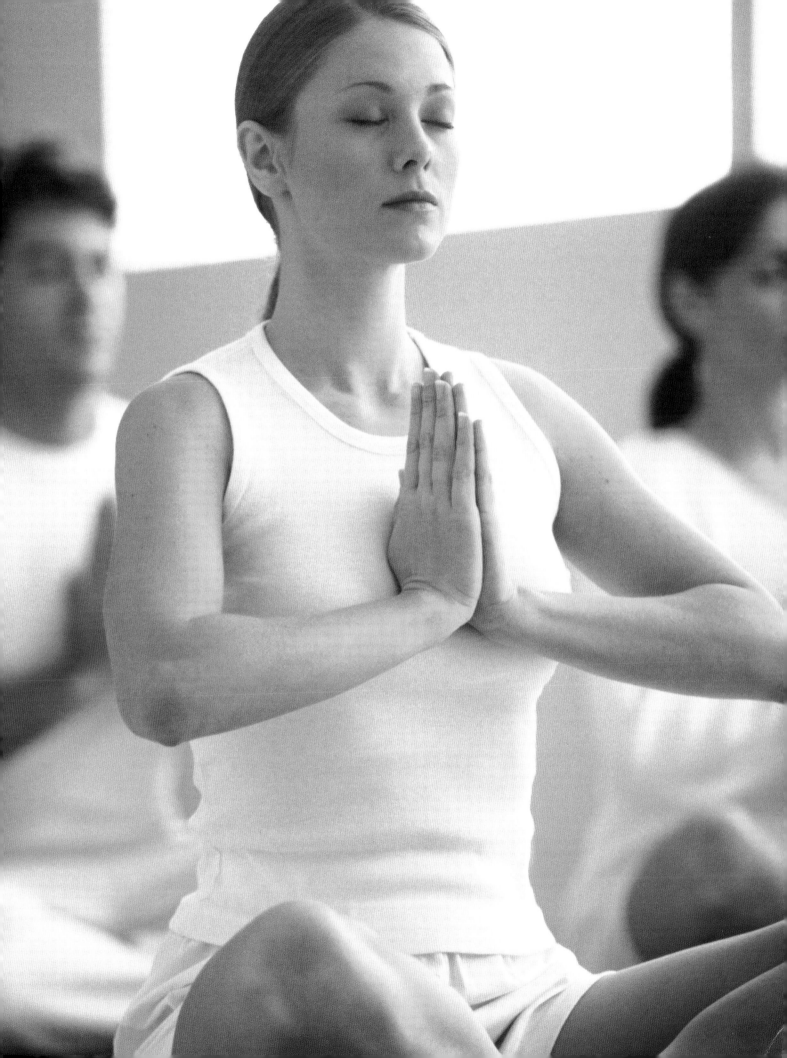

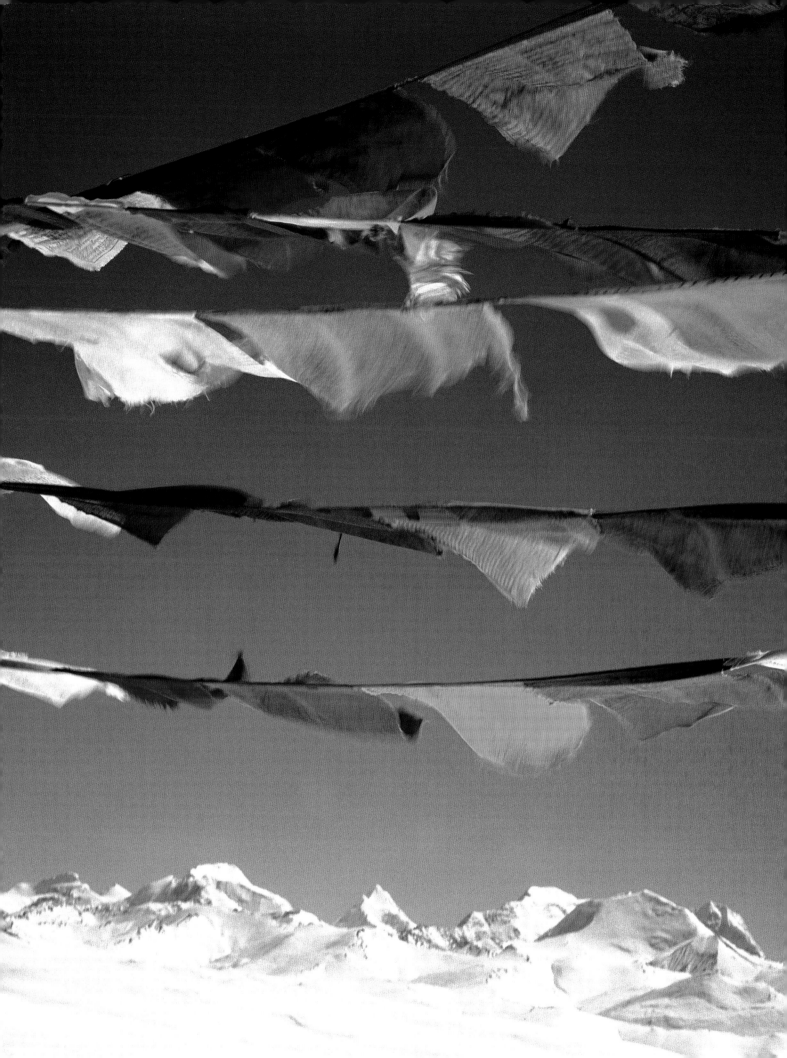

# the benefits of meditation

You want to beat stress and relax? Boost your concentration and sharpen your brain? Alleviate a chronic ailment like insomnia? Stop being angry or just be a nicer person? Meditation is the answer.

## stress release

We all need a shot of adrenaline and cortisol (stress hormones) in the system to get things done—if we had no sense of urgency and heightened reflexes, we'd never meet deadlines or manage to cross the road safely. Stress hormones are released in response to a perceived threat or demand. They cause blood pressure to rise, muscle tension to increase, the heart to beat faster, and the breathing to become more rapid and shallow. All this equips the body to respond to the threat or demand by running away or fighting. Modern inventions such as cell phones and e-mail mean you can never get away from demands that cause stress hormones to be released. When we don't act to relieve the tension that the hormones cause to build up over a period of time, the elevated blood pressure and heart rate, changes to breathing, and movement of blood to muscles leads to ill health. Stress has now replaced back pain as the biggest cause of absenteeism from work.

Meditation eases stress-related symptoms. A study in the 1960s by Dr. Herbert Benson at Harvard Medical School showed that meditation returns stress hormone levels to normal, relaxes the muscles, and slows the heart rate. In short, meditation induces a relaxation response that reduces mental anxiety and physical tension.

## calmness and inner quiet

Meditation offers more than this sheer relaxation, blissful though it is. It brings about an inner stillness and clarity of awareness that can introduce a spiritual dimension to life. When you meditate, you start to appreciate a special or sacred—some might say divine—quality to everything. For its ability to bring this about, meditation is integral to the world's major religious traditions.

## reduced negativity

Meditation is an antidote to difficult emotions such as anger and jealousy. Techniques urge you to stand back and watch yourself in everyday situations until you become aware of your habitual reactions. Like seeing yourself on a video, this can make for uncomfortable viewing. As you meditate more and more, you gain an understanding of why you act like you do. This self-awareness prompts you to stop as you start to get angry and get rid of habits that make you feel bad about yourself. Specific techniques show how to temper and harness these difficult emotions to harvest good from bad.

## focused concentration

By putting your brain into neutral with meditation, you give it a well-earned rest. When your mind is clear of clutter, you can discern what's important and easily discard what isn't. Suddenly your thinking sharpens, your concentration span lengthens, and you become more efficient and incisive. You know what your priorities are and find it easier to plan to achieve them. In studies, people who meditate report increased performance and greater job satisfaction at work, and students report an improved ability to study and retain information, leading to better academic achievement.

**left:** In Tibet, breezes carry the meditative thoughts inscribed on Buddhist prayer flags to the heavens.

## instant energy

Alongside the calmness and insight of meditation comes renewed vitality and enthusiasm. It can feel strongly exhilarating to meditate. The breath and mind-control techniques refresh the brain and body after a long day, act as an instant energy blast at work, and, when you learn to bring mindful awareness into every activity, recharge you as you go about the day.

## living in the present

Meditation isn't confined to one place and time; you can use the techniques to bring a meditative awareness to everything you do, from showering to strength training, simply by staying aware of every action and letting go of intrusive thoughts. The more you live consciously in the present, the more you free your mind from polluting emotions such as guilt and regret about the past and anticipation of the uncertain future. And so you relax. From this detached place of clarity, calm, and focus, you can respond in a more measured and appropriate way to people and events. When you live in the now, you also experience life to the fullest: with an uncluttered mind, you really see the colors of autumn leaves, appreciate a lover, focus on a book or piece of music, and taste good food. By allowing you to see what's important and get the most out of every moment, meditation helps you simplify your home and work affairs, your belongings, and your social life.

## freedom for all

Living in the present liberates you from worry, fear, and attachment to things that will inevitably break, get lost, or move away. You get a glimpse of what it's like to live in the flow, aware of everything but unphased by it, broad in perspective, serene, and free from suffering. Many meditation techniques show ways to extend this clarity of awareness to help other people. By developing compassion, love, and kindness, meditation helps you help others.

# how meditation works

Unless you're a practiced yogi, your mind is all over the place most of the time. As you perform a simple task, such as brushing your teeth, your brain is assaulted by a thousand thoughts as well as the job at hand. As I write this, I'm planning to go pick tomatoes from the garden, craving a sandwich, trying to remember whether my daughter's soccer clothes are clean, anticipating questions for the journalist interviewing me tomorrow, worrying that the baby will wake and keep me from working, and reviewing yesterday's yoga class. As I get caught up in all this, my breathing becomes shallow, my heart pounds, and I lose focus. Meditation stops this.

Meditation induces a state of relaxed alertness or thoughtless awareness. As you bring attention to one focus—a word or picture, perhaps, or the movement of breath in and out—the mind gently rests, suspending thought. The more you practice, the longer the gap between thoughts.

## picturing meditation

Measuring electrical activity in the brain with an electroencephalograph (EEG) gives a visual image of brain wave patterns. From this, we can see what the state of meditation looks like. Brain waves produced when we sleep, dream, or are awake differ from each other. Waking brain waves are typically fast. The state of deep sleep shows an increased frequency in alpha waves—those associated with quiet relaxation and receptivity—indicating that the body is relaxing and the nervous system that reverses the fight-or-flight stress response (the parasympathetic system) is taking control.

Research reveals that the alpha wave level is much higher during meditation than in sleep and that, unlike in sleep, intensity is evenly synchronized across both hemispheres of the brain: the dominant side that governs rational and logical functions and the nondominant side, associated with creativity and emotional responses. This synchronizing of brain waves between the left and right sides of the cortex, the largest part of the brain, has been shown to optimize brain functioning and boost IQ scores. Other studies have shown that blood flow in the brain is boosted during meditation.

That meditation is better at relaxing accumulated stress and tension than sleep or any leisure activity has been supported by many research studies since the 1960s. Participants in trials report that meditation makes them feel calmer and more relaxed, and simultaneously more alert, focused, and efficient, improving performance at work and school and increasing job satisfaction scores.

## the mind/body link

A growing proportion of the medical establishment is becoming convinced by mounting evidence that when the mind is relaxed, the body seems to be less susceptible to disease and better able to heal itself. Research since the 1980s has explored the role of the emotions in stimulating neuropeptides, chemical messengers in the nervous system, to affect the functioning of body systems as diverse as the digestive and immune systems. When the brain experiences feelings of calmness and happiness, for example, the production of neuropeptides (endorphins, the body's natural opiates, are one) seems to trigger a lowering of blood pressure and the relaxation of muscles—physical relaxation. It seems you can think yourself into relaxation at will, a fact well documented over the last 5,000 years by people who meditate.

# meditation and health

Hundreds of medical studies prove the health benefits of meditation. Research demonstrates that people who meditate visit the doctor less often. They have lower cholesterol and blood pressure levels, less incidence of heart disease and depression, and take fewer days off work than people who don't meditate; they also report a better body image and self-confidence. Meditation has also been shown to have remarkable healing powers for those who suffer ill health, from migraines and irritable bowels to heart disease. Such striking data has lead some family doctors to prescribe meditation as the first treatment of choice for some conditions.

## stress and illness

Stressful emotions are linked with a higher risk of ill health: some 80–90 percent of illnesses are thought to be connected with stress. Experiencing stress seems to repress the immune system, reducing the production of antibodies and T cells. Students have been shown to be more likely to suffer colds at times of stress; for example, when taking exams. By changing the way you think and relaxing completely using meditation, you can protect against disease and help treat illnesses by boosting the immune system. A 1993 Canadian study shows a 70 percent increase in immune-strengthening beta endorphins following meditation.

## meditation for long life

Meditating seems to keep the effects of aging at bay. Studies of people who use Transcendental Meditation show that they have a biological age significantly lower than their chronological age, with mental, physical, cognitive, and perceptual abilities equivalent to those of much younger people. They live longer, too. This has been linked with the fact that people who meditate seem to maintain levels of a hormone (dehydroepiandrosterone sulfate, or DHEA-S) that decreases with age. Low levels have been associated with disease and mortality. Transcendental Meditators share levels with people up to ten years their junior.

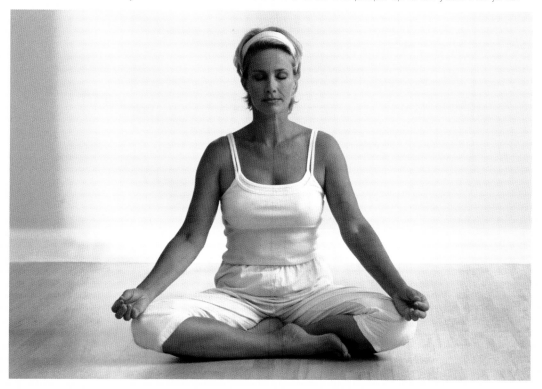

## meditation and specific diseases

Note: Most research into the health benefits of meditation is based on Transcendental Meditation (TM).

---

**Chronic illness** Meditation is supremely effective at tackling the range of debilitating illnesses that conventional Western medicine finds difficult to diagnose and treat. Migraine and tension headaches, insomnia, irritable bowel syndrome, and premenstrual syndrome have been shown to respond well to meditation. In a 2001 study, asthma patients using Sahaja yoga meditation showed improvement in breathing patterns and more responsiveness to medication (equivalent to an extra dose) than those using relaxation techniques.

---

**Pain care** Meditation can help people live with chronic pain, as well as release some of the muscle tension that contributes to the pain cycle. Patients in pain clinics who used mind/body relaxation techniques reported less depression and anxiety and reduced their number of visits to the doctor for treatment by 39 percent. People who meditate have been shown to recover more speedily from surgery and spend 50 percent less time in the hospital than those who don't.

---

**High blood pressure** TM was shown to be more effective than either relaxation or regular treatment plans at rapidly reducing systolic and diastolic pressure levels for men and women (it seems to keep blood vessels open). Being without side effects and easy to continue at home, meditation is routinely recommended by doctors to those at risk from stroke.

---

**Heart disease** Dr. Dean Ornish was able to reverse coronary heart disease in a 1992 study using a program that included meditation. Patients with angina pectoris who practiced TM showed significant improvement in their ability to exercise and to continue for longer periods at a higher intensity than a control group.

---

**Cancer care** Therapy programs to complement medical treatment often include meditation. It can reduce unpleasant symptoms that accompany chemotherapy treatment. Cancer patients using behavioral intervention techniques such as meditation report improved quality of life, reduced pain, and less psychological distress. In two studies, cancer patients who meditated survived for twice as long as those who did not.

---

**Mental health** A 1992 report showed that Buddhist Vipassana meditation could reduce anxiety, agoraphobia, and panic attacks. Other reports reveal that meditation is effective in relieving mild depression, hostility, and emotional instability. One 2001 British study showed that patients who practiced meditation improved more than those receiving behavioral therapy alone. Patients with post-traumatic stress responded markedly better to TM than to standard psychotherapy treatments. People with post-traumatic stress disorder and depression commonly show a reduction in the size of the hippocampus (the part of the brain that deals with emotions and instincts and is associated with the stress hormone cortisol), perhaps caused by increased levels of cortisol. PET scans of the brain show that meditation increases activity in the hippocampus.

---

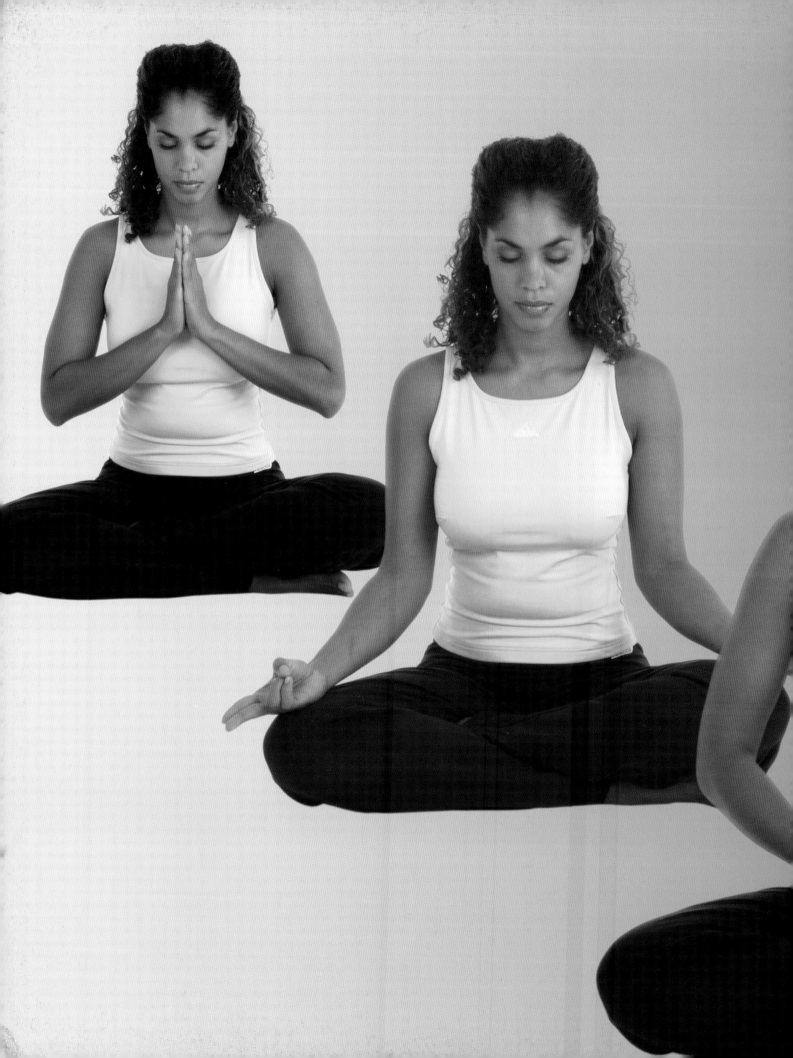

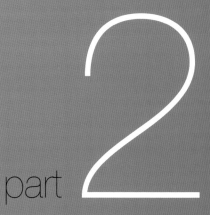

part 2

starting to
meditate

# preparing the space

It makes sense to try to set aside a special space at home for your meditation practice; it could be no more than three feet square, but should be a quiet sanctuary, tucked away from the pressures of everyday life, and ideally light, airy, and with a view. You might even prefer to choose a spot outdoors. Meditating in one spot seems to charge the space with good vibes, which augment with practice. Above all, your tranquillity zone should feel welcoming and calming the moment you step over the threshold. Try not to use your meditation space for other activities.

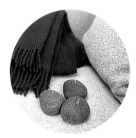

## cleansing the space

First, clear the clutter. Nothing muddies your thinking as much as distracting objects. As most people sit on the floor to meditate, it's also important to keep your meditation space clean and dust-free. Indeed, Tibetan spiritual teachers state that the first stage to enlightenment is sweeping the meditation area clean. To purify the space further, add three or four drops of purifying and sense-quickening rosemary, lemongrass, or eucalyptus oil to the final rinse water when mopping the floor. You might also like to charge the space with energy-cleansing techniques for ultimate good vibes. Chime a pair of tiny finger cymbals at the corners of the room, visualizing negative energy disappearing as you do so, and sprinkle a few drops of rose water over the floor. Use a blessing from your own faith tradition as you work, if desired. Chanting "Om" (page 119) is thought to clear and purify the meditation space. Always remove your shoes before entering the space to keep it physically and energetically clean, and repeat the cleansing rituals whenever you feel stuck in your meditation.

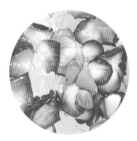

## the essentials

Personalize your space with a beautiful rug and a few special cushions to place beneath your legs and knees as you learn to kneel or sit cross-legged. You might like to look for a traditional Japanese circular zafu meditation cushion used in the Zen zazen tradition (Tibetan cushions are square). Some people prefer to work on a firm futon on the floor. You will also need a comfortable shawl or blanket (a soft pashmina blanket is perfect) to guard against cold. If you plan to practice yoga, you'll also need a yoga mat.

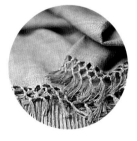

## a home altar

Some people who meditate like to create an altar in the meditation space. It might be modest and informal—just a bunch of fresh flowers or a lit candle on a low table or shelf. Or it could be faith-based, centered around a sacred statue or symbol—perhaps the Blessed Virgin, Star of David, Lord Ganesha, or the Buddha—with offerings of flowers, food, incense, or candles. Don't be put off if you have no faith tradition. Use an altar to reflect your personality and display what inspires you: treasures picked up on nature walks, such as seashells, pinecones, and leaves; glitzy sequins and rhinestones; family photos; and poetic quotes.

## spiritually uplifting scents

**frankincense:** deepens breathing, enhances calmness, helps bring about a state conducive to prayer

**bergamot:** spirit-lifting and mood-enhancing

**cypress:** purifying and aids deep breathing; an ancient symbol of eternal life (avoid during pregnancy)

**jasmine:** lethargy-busting antidepressant (avoid during pregnancy)

**juniper:** air-purifying and calming (avoid during pregnancy)

**melissa (true):** uplifting, restorative for the emotions

**sandalwood:** spiritually therapeutic scent; considered meditation-enhancing since Vedic times

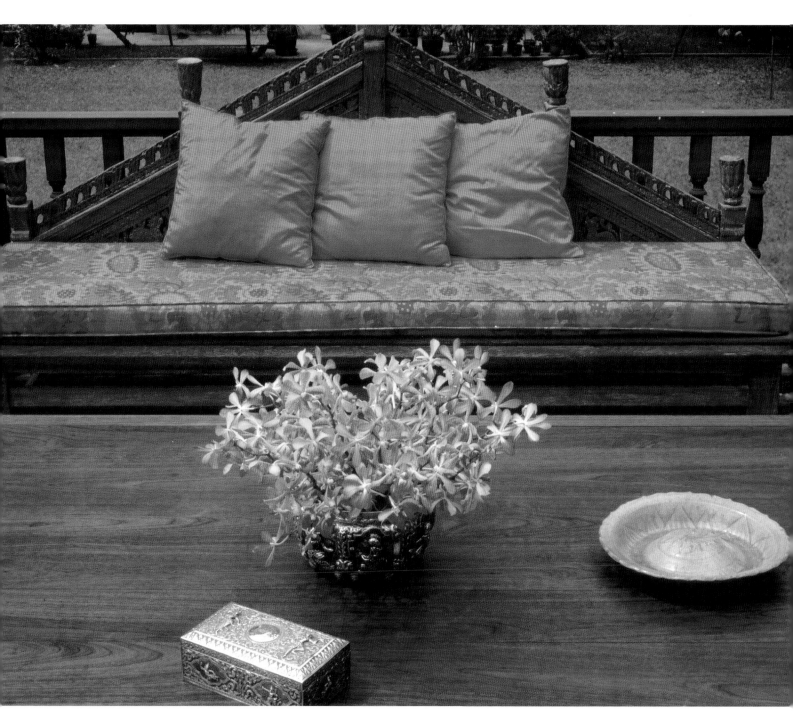

## scenting the space

Some scents have a long history of association with the ceremony of inner journeying: frankincense, for example, has been shown to heighten the effects of meditation by deepening the breathing, calming the mind, and restoring emotional balance. Choose spiritually uplifting scents from those listed on the left to burn as incense or use in essential-oil vaporizers—add two to four drops to the water bowl—or make an air freshener by dropping two drops of essential oil into a plant sprayer. Shake well, then spritz the room.

## where in the home?

Vaastu, the art of interior design often referred to as "Indian feng shui," recommends the northeastern sector of your home as the best place for a meditation or yoga tranquillity zone. Prana, life's energy, is thought to emanate from the northeast, and enters a home from this point on the compass.

# sitting positions

Meditation is best practiced sitting in a comfortable position with the spine upright—as if supporting the sky with your head. For some people this means full Lotus Pose with feet resting on the opposite thigh; for others it means sitting on a straight-backed chair with feet flat on the floor. The fundamental is that the position is so comfortable that you don't start wriggling or slouching after a couple of minutes. When you are physically stable, it becomes easier to enter the meditative state.

## positions to try

Play with the poses here to find one that suits you, then work with it for some time before progressing to a more difficult sitting position. Sukhasana is the easiest and most stable pose for beginners; the full Lotus Pose is the most challenging. If you start to slouch in any posture or find yourself wriggling with pain, return to an easier pose. Make sure you vary the crossing of the legs each time you practice.

## sukhasana  easy pose

❶ Sit on the floor with legs stretched wide. Pull the flesh out from behind your buttocks, then sit upright. Fold one leg in so the heel sits next to the opposite inner thigh.

❷ Bend the other leg and draw the lower leg in, tucking the foot beneath the opposite shin in a crossed-leg position. Let both knees relax down to the floor. Rest your hands on your thighs or knees, or in one of the mudra hand gestures (pages 26–27).

❸ Pull your spine up and out of your pelvis, lengthening the crown of the head away from the base of the spine, chin in and parallel to the floor, back of the neck long. Pull your abdominal muscles in and up to support the spine.

## siddhasana   **perfect pose**

❶ Sit on the floor with legs stretched wide. Pull the flesh out from behind your buttocks, then sit upright. Fold one leg in so the heel sits next to your pubic bone, the sole by the inside of the opposite thigh.

❷ Bend the other leg and draw the lower leg in, placing the foot on top of the lower foot, ankles and heels stacked. Gently rest your hands on your thighs or knees, or in one of the mudra hand gestures (pages 26–27), and lengthen the spine as in Sukhasana.

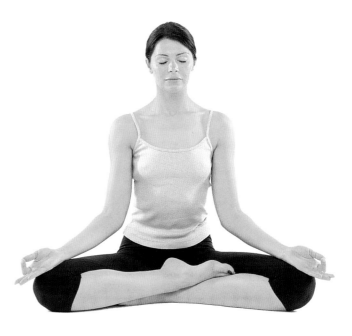

## padmasana   **lotus pose (including half-lotus)**

❶ Sit on the floor with legs stretched wide. Pull the flesh out from behind your buttocks, then sit upright. Bend the left leg, taking the foot against the right thigh near the groin.

❷ Bend the right leg. Support the foot with both hands and place it on the left thigh, outer edge by the groin, sole up—this is the Half-lotus Pose. Practice with each leg for some weeks before bringing the left foot over the right knee onto the right thigh, outer edge near the groin, sole up—the full Lotus Pose.

❸ Rest the hands on the thighs or knees or in a mudra. Extend the spine and sides of the torso up and out of the pelvis, lengthening the back of the neck and feeling the crown of the head pulling toward the ceiling. Breathe into areas of discomfort and release tension with each out breath.

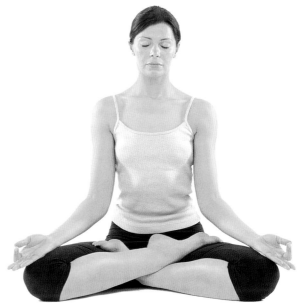

### why sit upright?

On a purely physical level, keeping the back upright opens the chest and gives room for the diaphragm to move, allowing maximum oxygen to enter the body on the in breath and enabling full exhalation on the out breath. This increases alertness. It may also be a throwback to times when prayer was performed standing up, the body acting as a physical conductor linking the spirit realm with the earth. Sitting with spine erect but legs folded keeps that connection but enables longer periods of meditation.

Yoga theory maintains that when the spine is upright, subtle life energy, prana, can pass up the body's main energy channel, the sushumna, which runs alongside the spine from the energy reservoir sited at the base. As prana moves up toward the crown of the head, it invigorates every part of the body and expands the mind by activating powerful energy centers, chakras. Establishing a firm seat with certain sitting postures enables the spine to remain straight.

# sitting on a chair

If you have real difficulties sitting on the floor, don't struggle with it—use a firm, hard-backed chair instead. When you can easily hold yourself upright on the chair for twenty minutes, try the floor sitting positions again. This is also a good way to grab a couple of minutes' meditation in the office or in a parked car.

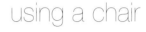

## using a chair

❶ Choose a hard-backed chair with a firm seat, such as a dining chair. Remove your shoes in order to make yourself more stable. Sit on the seat so that the backs of both thighs are supported but well in front of the back of the chair.

❷ Place both feet flat on the floor, making a right angle with your knees. If both feet don't reach flat to the floor, place blocks or piles of books beneath them until they do, planting your heels directly beneath your knees. Make sure your shoulders are directly above your hips, and rest your hands on your thighs or knees.

❸ Extend the spine and sides of the torso up and out of the pelvis equally on both sides. Lengthen out the dip in the lower back by drawing the abdominal muscles in, and extend the back of the neck, chin tucked in and parallel to the floor. Imagine you are suspended by a string from the crown of your head.

# kneeling positions

In some meditation systems, kneeling is preferred. When the buttocks rest on the ankles, a position known in yoga as Vajrasana, or the Thunderbolt Pose, the body feels grounded and powerful and a sense of serenity fills the mind. Virasana takes the pose one stage further. With each position, work toward the point at which you can keep the body still for some time; when the body is motionless, the mind can be too. Breathe into discomfort to lessen it.

## vajrasana thunderbolt pose

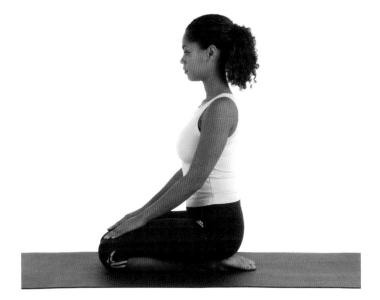

❶ Kneel with feet and ankles touching, knees together, hips over knees, shoulders over hips, toes pointing away. Sit back, pressing your buttocks down on your heels. Rest your hands on your knees or thighs.

❷ Take your focus to your legs and feet. Let your body weight sink down through your pelvis and inhale space into the lower legs, letting go of tightness and tension with the exhalation. Let your weight flatten out your feet and ankles.

❸ Lengthen your spine, opening the chest and releasing the shoulders. Tuck the chin in and release the back of the skull up from the back of the neck, head pulling toward the ceiling.

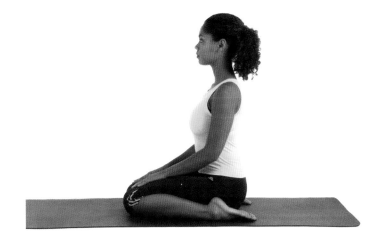

## virasana hero pose

❶ Kneel with knees together, hips over knees, shoulders over hips, toes pointing away. Sit back, letting your buttocks drop between your calves to rest on the floor. Make sure the outer thighs and calves remain touching.

❷ Breathe space into the legs and knees and extend up and out of the pelvis as before, working to reduce the curve in the lower back. Feel the weight of your buttocks bearing downward as your head extends toward the ceiling.

## using props

If you feel particularly inflexible or uncomfortable after sitting or kneeling for ten minutes or more, use cushions to aid the pose. When sitting in Sukhasana or Siddhasana, wedge a cushion in under your sitting bones and place more cushions beneath your knees. Place yoga blocks or paperback books under your feet if they don't touch the floor when you sit on a chair. In Vajrasana, place a cushion under your knees and buttocks or between your ankles. In Virasana, put a cushion under your buttocks.

# hand positions

Resting the backs of the hands on the knees or thighs with palms up has a physiological purpose: it keeps the shoulders and neck relaxed to aid extension of the spine. In many traditions it also has a spiritual function and is thought to affect your inner world. Mudras, or hand positions, activate the energy channels known as nadis in the Indian tradition and meridians in traditional Chinese medicine, as well as energy points, or acupoints, along them. This creates a closed circuit of subtle energy that keeps the prana life force from escaping from the mind/body circuit (the Sanskrit word *mudra* means "sealing" or "closure").

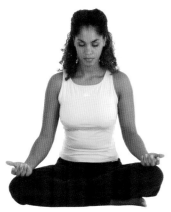

## palms up

To open yourself up to circulating energy, rest the back of your hands on your knees or thighs, palms up and fingers relaxed.

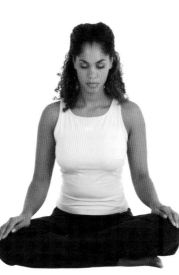

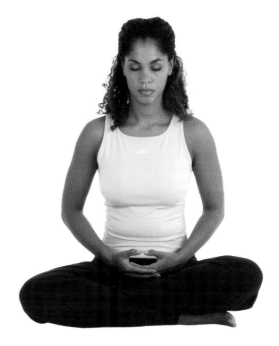

## palms down

To increase your sense of security and grounding, place your palms flat against your knees or thighs.

## cosmic mudra

### bowing

After some forms of practice, such as zazen in Zen Buddhism or after some yoga practice, one is expected to bow. This shows an effort to reduce your own status and self-centered focus. Give this a try. To those who feel least able to do it, bowing is considered most valuable, since you necessarily give up some of your pride in the act.

This is a common hand position for zazen meditation; it is also known as the meditation mudra.

Cup your hands in your lap close to your abdomen, palms up, left resting lightly on the right for women (reversed for men), middle joints of the middle finger aligned, thumbs barely touching to make an oval near your navel. Hold the arms lightly away from the body.

# jnana mudra

The traditional mudra symbolizing enlightenment, this hand position enables deep concentration and is said to activate the part of the brain associated with knowledge. It is also known as Vishnu mudra.

Stretch your palms and fingers out, then rest your hands, palms upward, loosely on your knees. Bring the tips of the first finger and thumb on each hand to touch lightly. Stretch out your three remaining digits, fingers touching.

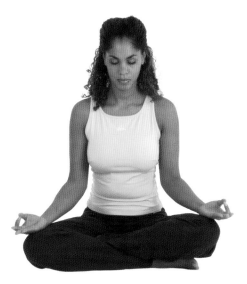

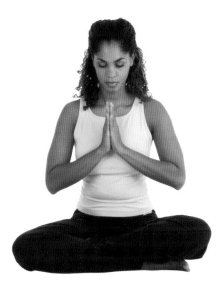

# namaskar mudra

The fingers make a steeple pointing toward the heavens in this cross-cultural gesture of prayer and humility. When the palms and thumbs are opened slightly, it becomes a Buddhist sign of offering; when the fingers are opened like a fan, Christians see themselves opening up to divine love. It may also be called the prostration mudra.

Bring both palms and fingers together in front of your chest, pressing each digit into its opposite and making contact with every part of each palm. Press your thumbs lightly into your sternum, opening your chest, shoulders relaxed and dropping away from your ears.

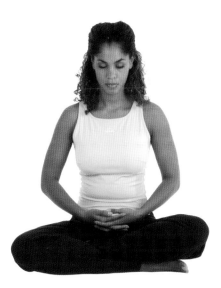

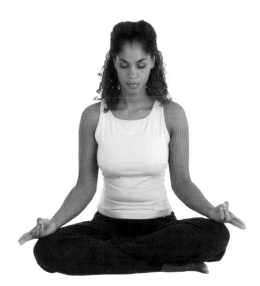

# prana mudra

To promote the free flow of prana energy for ultimate well-being, bend the ring and little fingers toward the palm and secure them lightly with the tip of the thumb. Straighten the index and middle fingers.

# gomukha mudra

To represent the coming together of body and mind, interlink the fingers and thumbs and cup the hands lightly in your lap, close to your abdomen.

# lying down

Many schools of meditation warn against meditating while lying down—you can easily drift off to sleep; this is not the aim of meditation! However, relaxing the body by lying down is a good way to relinquish tension from mind and body before starting actual meditation. It can also be a good way to reflect in bed last thing at night, and it suits those with health problems that preclude sitting upright for long periods. The exercise below stills each part of the body in turn in yoga's most important and, though motionless, most difficult posture, Savasana, or the Corpse Pose.

## total body relaxation in savasana

❶ Lie on your back on a yoga mat or blanket. Bend your knees, feet flat on the floor. Take a few breaths and feel your sacrum (the back of the pelvis) widen and sink into the ground. Extend each leg so they lie slightly apart, feet falling outward, while maintaining the heaviness of the sacrum. Relax your arms away from your body, palms up. Lift your head to make sure it is aligned with the body, and relax it back down to the floor. Close your eyes.

❷ Tense and relax every part of the body in turn, starting with the feet. Tense the left foot, screwing up the toes, and release to the floor. Repeat with the right foot. Tense the left calf, knee, and thigh, tightening the muscles as much as possible, then let them drop to the floor. Repeat on the right.

❸ Clench your buttocks, lifting them from the ground, then release. Press the sacrum and legs to the floor. Now imagine all the tension running down your lower body and out through your toes.

❹ Screw up your face, jaw, mouth, eyes, and forehead. Release. Widen your mouth, eyes, and ears; flare your nostrils. Release. Imagine the tension flowing out through the crown of your head. Feel your jaw loose, tongue relaxed, teeth set apart. Relax your nose, each eye and ear, smooth your brow, let the scalp melt, and feel the skin on the back of your head melt into the floor.

❺ Pull in the abdomen, holding the breath as long as possible, then release. Tense the muscles of the chest, then relax. Make a fist with the left hand, extend your straightened fingers, then let them drop. Repeat on the other hand. Straighten and tense the entire left arm, then release. Repeat on the other side.

❻ Tighten the shoulders and neck, pressing the chin into the chest, then let everything drop. Feel every part of your torso melting into the floor. Visualize all the tension running down your arms and spine and seeping out of your body at your tailbone and fingertips.

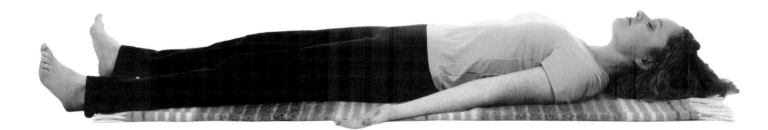

❼ Sense each part of the body to ensure it is still relaxed. Command any awkward areas—the back of the waist, the back of the neck—to become heavy and sink into the floor. Then focus inside on your breathing, feeling it quiet and deepen.

❽ Remain in the pose for ten minutes or longer; sense every part of your body completely relaxed and yet tingling with energy. Try not to drift into sleep; instead, continue sensing your body for tension and visualize it dissolving. Then wriggle your fingers and toes, gently open your eyes, stretch, turn onto your right side, and take a few minutes to rise.

## using props

If you have lower back problems, place a cushion beneath your knees. If you have difficulty in breathing easily with your head on the floor, support your head and upper back with firm pillows to open the chest and raise the diaphragm.

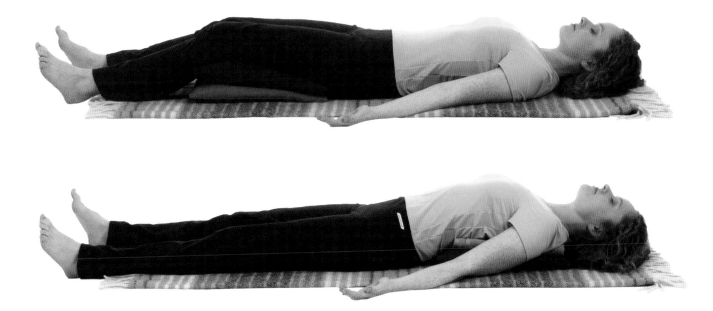

# breathwork

Breathing is the essential tool of meditation since the act always takes place in the present. Taking your attention to your breathing immediately removes it from the convoluted machinations of the mind and emotions and into the now. Yogis teach that when you inhale, you take within you prana, a Sanskrit word that means not just "breath," but also the energy of the universe: in breathing, you connect with the essence of life and everything outside you. Use the breathing techniques set out here to start exploring your breathing patterns.

## the mind/body link

The act of breathing is so entwined with the body, nervous system, and functioning of the brain that thought patterns alone can cause breathing to change and affect physiological functioning—think how anger or anxiety result in shallow breathing, a racing heart, and the inability to think clearly.

Conversely, consciously slowing and deepening the breath slows down the heart rate, allows adequate oxygen to nourish every part of the body, and restores mental and emotional equanimity. Calming a restless mind is as easy as deepening and quieting your breathing.

## learning to feel the breath

❶ Sit comfortably upright, either on the floor with legs crossed and back straight, or on an upright chair, feet flat on the ground (pages 22–24). Place your hands low over your abdomen, fingertips touching.

❷ As you breathe in, bypass your chest and shoulders and feel the air drop toward the abdomen, causing your fingertips to draw away from each other. Visualize inflating a balloon in your abdomen from the bottom up. Notice how the back of your waist and rib cage subtly expand.

❸ As you exhale, visualize the air leaving your abdominal area little by little from the top down and notice your fingertips touch again.

❹ Keep the image of the balloon expanding and deflating, but take your focus to your nostrils and the flow of breath in and out, feeling it cooling your upper lip and expanding the lower part of your nostrils. Work for three to five minutes, watching your breath gradually lengthen and become deeper.

### reconnecting with the breath

Train yourself to reconnect with your breathing whenever you remember during the day. At first you might want to set an alarm on your cell phone or watch to jog your memory; soon it will become habitual. Your breath is the one constant in your life. Bringing your awareness to it allows you to reconnect with yourself and the present at any time and in any situation. Whether you work for a few seconds or a few minutes, this gives you refreshing space to step outside the tangled web of thoughts, emotions, and concerns that defines everyday life, and to break cycles of thought and action that lead nowhere.

## quick breath check

Place one palm on your chest, the other flat on your abdomen. Without changing your regular breathing pattern, notice which hand moves. If it's the upper hand, you're breathing shallowly: a very common problem that restricts the flow of breath, can lead to muscle tension in the chest, neck, and shoulders, and can cause digestive problems. Use the "Learning to Feel the Breath" exercise on the previous page to improve the way you breathe.

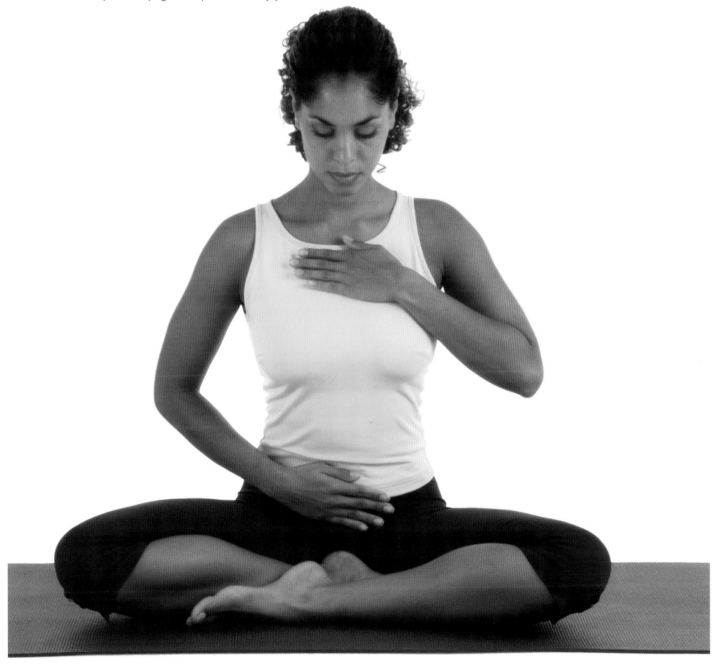

# essential techniques

Here is advice on when, how often, and how long to practice meditation. The most important thing to remember is to take it slowly and release your mind from worrying about getting somewhere. Even if you never reach the stage at which you can maintain focused attention for seconds, let alone minutes, simply witnessing the distraction of your restless mind and its constant stream of disconnected thoughts is a step forward.

### what to wear
Loose, comfortable clothing is best; anything that doesn't restrict around the waist and chest or distract your mind. As you sit still and meditate, your heart rate slows and the body cools. After a yoga session or other form of exercise, this will seem even more marked, so add a shawl or sweatshirt and socks before you start to meditate. Always take off your shoes, the better to connect with earth energy and also to remove yourself from thoughts of the outside world.

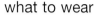

### when to practice
The quiet of early morning is a good time for meditation—especially for busy people whose days race away with them. It helps set your default for the day into a calm, unflustered, giving mode. Get up before the rest of your household to ensure you're not interrupted. Work toward adding another session just before bed to wind down and release the day's preoccupations before sleep.

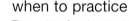

### when not to practice
Many people slump in the midafternoon and early evening, so these might not be the best times to start your meditation practice, as it could turn into a nap. Don't meditate immediately after eating: the digestive process can make you feel drowsy and the abdomen may not feel comfortable.

### how often
Some days meditation seems easier than on others. Sometimes everything flows and meditation is effortless. Other times, the minutes drag, you get an uncontrollable urge to scratch or wriggle, and your mind stays stuck in overdrive. The secret is not to try too hard and not to start with set expectations.

Start with three to five minutes, two or three times a week. Try to work in the same place at the same time of day. As you practice, you'll probably find that your commitment grows. Work gradually toward a twenty-minute session morning and evening, so you start and end the day relaxed and ready for anything.

### when to stop
Set the alarm on your cell phone, watch, alarm clock, or kitchen timer before you start meditating to avoid working in worried anticipation of the end. After finishing meditation, sit in silence for a while, becoming attuned to the outside world but retaining an inner awareness of composure, lack of worries, and peace.

## mindfulness 24/7
The more you meditate, the more you find yourself slipping into meditation mode as you carry out the regular tasks of everyday life. You bring "mindfulness" to your commute and your work, to washing up and changing the baby's diapers, to your sports performance, and to playtime with children. When you keep bringing your focus to the task at hand and inhabit it without thoughts of your next action or past memories, you have truly brought meditation into your life.

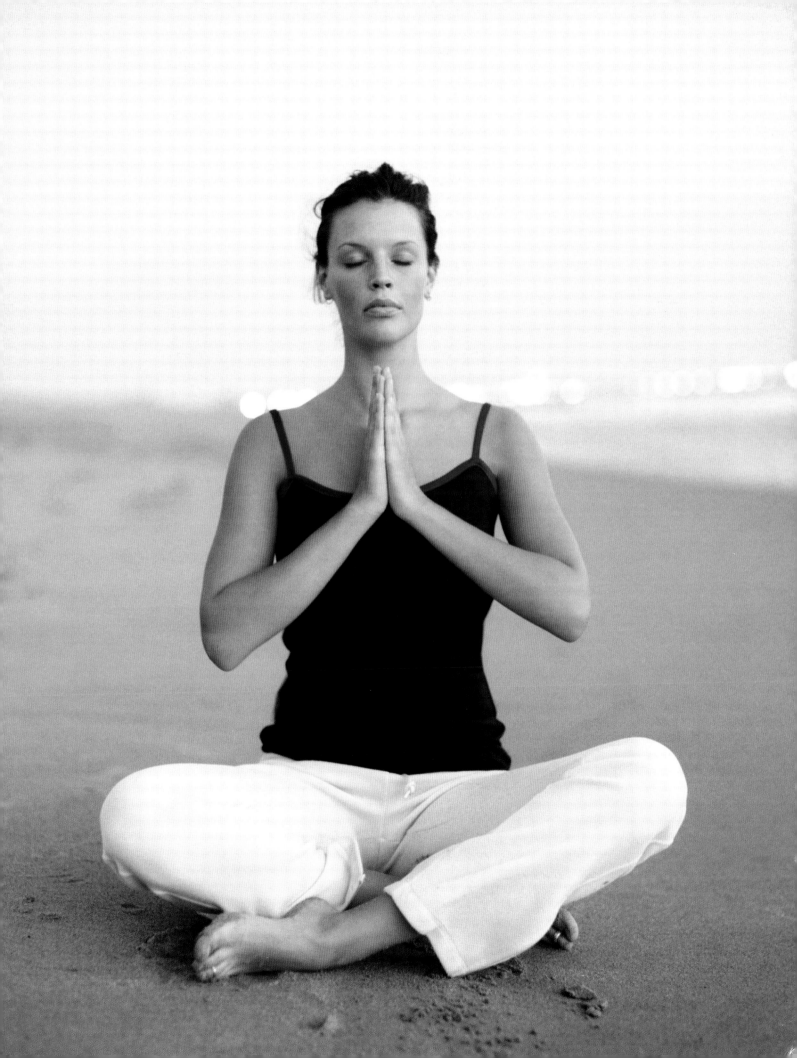

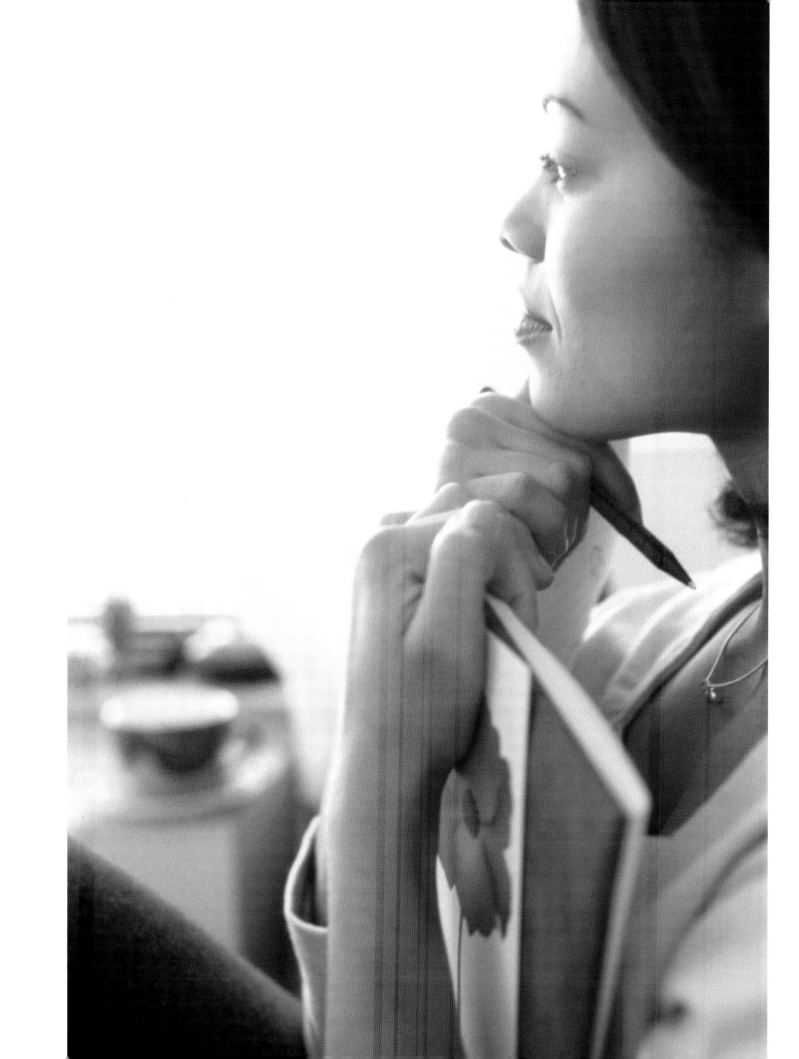

# basic meditation

This active technique allows you to start taking control of your response to events and thoughts by witnessing their effect on your body, mind, and emotions. Use the steps to learn that the essential you is not the you that reacts to outside events, but has a wider awareness of the big picture.

❶ Choose the sitting or kneeling position in which you feel most comfortable (pages 22–25) and relax your arms and hands (pages 26–27). Close your eyes. Take a few moments to release tension from your body: your feet, toes, and hands; your lower back, neck, and shoulders; and your forehead and jaw.

❷ Take your focus to your breathing. Feel the exhalation taking tension and toxins out of your body, and allow the in breath to come naturally. Let the breaths lengthen and become deeper without force of will or body. Don't control; just be aware of the breath coming in and out without you having to do anything.

❸ Draw your mind away from—and let go of—emotions that preoccupied you before you sat down. Push anger, anxiety, and boredom to one side and be at peace. Connect with the reasons that brought you to meditate today—perhaps a search for peace of mind, relaxation, or stress relief.

❹ Ask your brain to stop talking and switch off your intellect for a while. Imagine your mind as a blank screen. Watch thoughts and emotions pass onto the screen, then pass away again. Don't get involved in them. Turn off your urge to judge them and comment on or analyze them. Switch off your urge to follow their narrative.

❺ When, inevitably, you do find yourself following a train of thought, don't react or get angry or impatient, just take a step back and note the intricacy of the workings of your mind and wait for the screen to go blank again (which it will, given time). Alternatively, imagine light enveloping the thought or feeling and removing it like an eraser on a blackboard.

❻ When your time is up, slowly open your eyes, wriggle your fingers or toes, and take time to come to before getting up and going back to your daily activities.

## keeping a meditation journal

Keep a notebook and pen in your meditation space; then, after meditating, take a few minutes to record your experience. Note any difficulties or concerns and jot down the small achievements that keep you going. As you write and reread your entries, you may gain unexpected insight, be surprised by the patterns of disruptive thoughts, uncover transformative solutions, and gain fresh insight into what needs to change for you to progress.

## stilling thoughts

• When you find yourself following a train of thought or losing focus, return to the anchor of your constant breath moving in and out.

• Acknowledge that you have lost your focus, then return to the meditation without making judgments.

• Don't beat yourself up over losing focus. Be compassionate with yourself and try not to get hung up on perfection.

• Don't get overly confident, either: when you find yourself congratulating yourself on keeping your mind inactive, you have, naturally, drifted off course again.

• Witnessing what distracts you gives you insight, and so, oddly, is a step toward maintaining your focus.

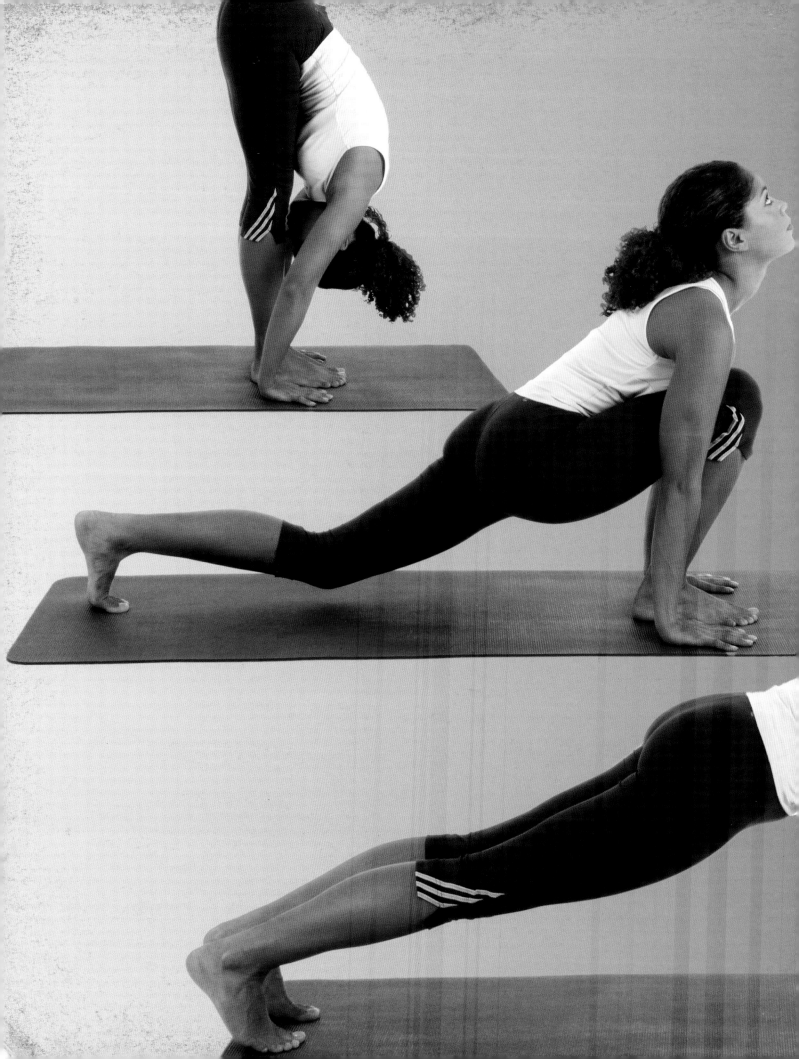

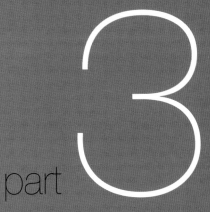

part 3

practical
meditations

"The supreme truth is established by total silence, not logical discussion and argument."
**Maharamayana**

# silent meditation

- **Just sitting**
- **Counting pebbles**
- **Breathing with beads**
- **Meditation with a candle**
- **Focusing on a flower**
- **Meditating with a spiritual object**
- **Mandala meditation**
- **Contemplating Celtic knotwork**
- **Zen puzzles**

Silence is a powerful tool in meditation: learning to sit still and quiet amid the incessant movement and noise that typifies modern living is a tough form of self-discipline and an increasingly rare skill. But surrendering to wordlessness is fundamental to finding out who you are. Sitting peacefully and in silence forces you to enter within and allows you to tune in to your innate sense of yourself and see what's happening right here, right now. Not for nothing do those on a spiritual quest make a vow of silence, from Lakota vision questers to Quakers. Zen masters teach that remaining absolutely motionless and silent in zazen sitting meditation is not just the route to enlightenment, it *is* enlightenment—the Buddha is described as being beyond "the paths of speech." Experiment with the meditations that follow: some employ a visual or intellectual focus, others bring about peace as you listen to nothing but the flow of breath and the beating of the heart.

# just sitting

The Zen term *zazen* translates as "just sitting," and that's all there is to this form of meditation at home. The Soto sect in Zen Buddhism considers that just sitting like the Buddha did when he achieved enlightenment is enlightenment itself. Teachers may suggest you use a focusing technique such as breathing or counting to bring the mind into the present (pages 112–13), but true zazen is the state you achieve when you are just being, aware of—but unfazed by—every sensation, thought, and emotion. Work for three to five minutes at first, building up to twenty minutes twice a day.

❶ Adopt a comfortable kneeling position (page 25). If you prefer, wedge a cushion beneath your buttocks to lessen the strain. Keep the spine erect, ears and shoulders aligned, and look ahead.

❷ Place your hands in Cosmic Mudra (page 26). Close your eyes halfway and focus forward and just down, softening your gaze. It helps to be facing a blank white wall to avoid visual distractions.

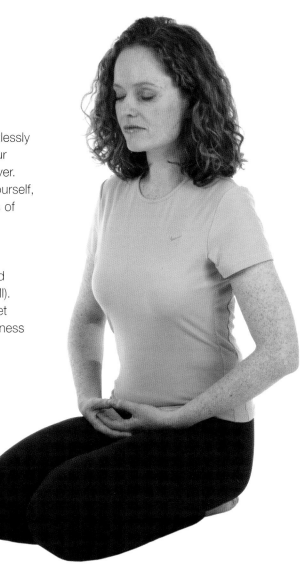

❸ Take your focus inside to watch your breath moving in and out effortlessly through your nostrils. Calmly move into witnessing mode, watching your thoughts, emotions, and sensations as if you are a disinterested observer. When a train of thoughts carries you away, as it will, do not chastise yourself, simply acknowledge it, ask it to pass through, and return to awareness of your breath moving in and out. Check your posture.

❹ When it's time to finish, come back to an awareness of the room and your body. Bow forward if you like (nine times in a zendo meditation hall). Wriggle your fingers and toes, then carefully unfold your legs. Sit in quiet reflection for a while before reentering the world, taking with you awareness of the peace and serenity you experienced during the sitting.

## when it hurts

Sitting in a posture for up to twenty minutes can be somewhat uncomfortable, even to those who have practiced meditation for many years. Make it your aim not to stop the discomfort, but to remain undisturbed by it. Being affected by aching legs but not being bothered reveals broadness of mind and tolerance.

## sitting right

Zen Master Shunryu Suzuki teaches that when you sit in the full Lotus Pose (page 23) for zazen, your left and right limbs become so entwined that you no longer know which is which. This interconnection is a physical symbol of the way in which the mind and body are one even while being separate. In zazen, to adopt a position is to inhabit the right state of mind. Those who can't easily achieve the final sitting or kneeling position often prove more adept at meditation: seeing imperfections and struggling with them often gives greater insight and makes for practitioners who are ever exploring and trying afresh to make a sincere effort.

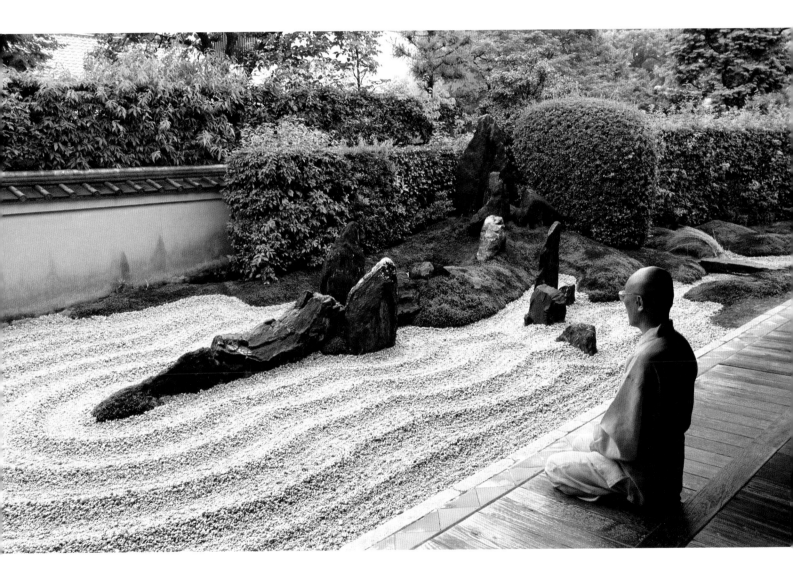

"After a heavy day at school, just sitting quietly with no noise makes me feel wonderful."

Alice, teacher

# counting pebbles

If you find the pure technique of zazen too intimidating, try this mindful counting exercise to give a focus to your silent meditation. Using a very physical focus such as pebbles anchors you to the here and now when the abstract nature of pure numbers is overwhelming. The desert fathers and mothers of the early Christian church are reputed to have counted pebbles from one pile to another to aid their silent contemplation. The practice also works to distract your attention when you're fretting over something. At home, keep about a dozen smooth pebbles, attractive stones, or marbles in a box specifically for this practice. Alternatively, work outdoors on a beach where pebbles can be found.

❶ Sit or kneel comfortably upright on the ground (pages 22–25). Pile up the pebbles in front of one knee.

❷ Take your focus inside, to your breath. Close your eyes at first if it helps. As you watch your breath moving in and out, let it wipe out other thoughts and all emotions.

❸ When you feel calm and steady, gently open your eyes and pick up the top pebble from the pile. Move it to one side to start a new pile, saying "one" silently and putting your complete focus on the stone.

❹ Repeat the action over and over, counting the pebbles silently from one pile to the other until the first pile is no more. Then start over. Work for up to five minutes, always allowing waves of thoughts that crash in to ebb away on their own as you take your focus back to the counting and the stones.

## counting your assets

At the end of a day, monks in parts of Tibet sit with two piles of pebbles: one black, one white. They are encouraged silently to review the day's events, rewarding themselves one white pebble for each act of kindness, one black pebble for each hurtful or uncaring action. You might keep two sets of pebbles, stones, or marbles to do the same. Don't overly chastise yourself each evening for another large pile of "bad" pebbles. Assess the piles over a longer time frame—a month, for example—to see whether the "good" pile gets bigger.

## bring it on

Although it's helpful for those new to meditation to start working with a physical focus, Zen teachers are happy when people lose their focus during meditation. If witnessing how changeable and fickle the mind is spurs you into more reflection and single-minded effort from the heart, you gain insight into the true nature of meditation and so progress faster than someone who flies through the techniques without seeing problems.

"In a year of meditating, I've never managed to keep my focus for even a few minutes, but I don't beat myself up over it because I still feel calmer and more relaxed than before."

**Howie, fitness instructor**

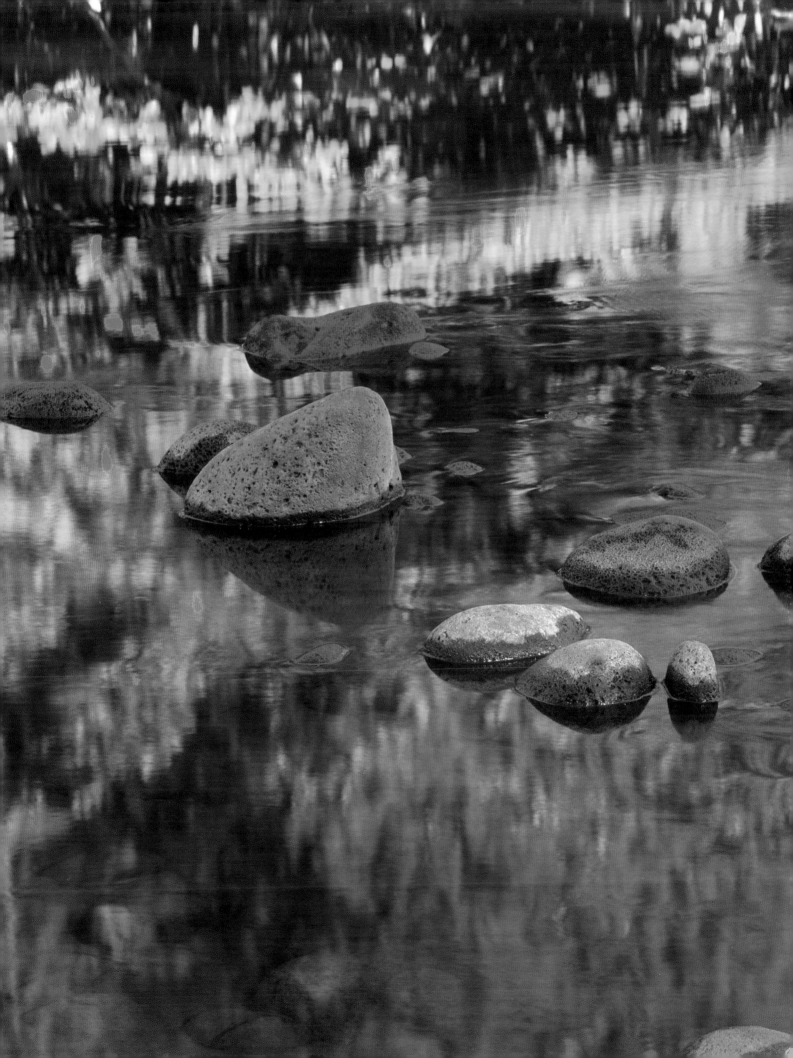

# breathing with beads

A prayer rope or thread of beads occupies a wandering mind and restless hands when you meditate to help you tune out of the world and into your heart. The mechanical act of passing each bead through your fingertips not only serves as a focus, it sets a helpful time limit on your meditation. For this breathing meditation you will need a rosary or mala, available from faith centers or New Age stores: those made of sandalwood or rose petals give off a meditation-enhancing scent when handled.

❶ Sit comfortably upright (pages 22–25), holding the prayer beads in your right hand by your heart. Take the first regular bead after the large introductory bead or chain between your middle finger and thumb. Close your eyes and center yourself by following your breath, feeling it lengthen and deepen.

❷ Inhale; as you exhale, roll the first bead between your middle finger and thumb. As you work, bring your total focus to the breath.

❸ Pass over each bead in the same way, linking the movement of your fingers with the rhythm of your lengthening in and out breaths. Each time your attention wavers, bring it back to the bead and the breath.

❹ When you reach the last bead, work back in the opposite direction. Do not cross the large bead. After finishing a full repetition forward and back, stop and sit in quiet contemplation for a few minutes or repeat more cycles of repetition (Buddhists and Hindus might aim for the auspicious number 108).

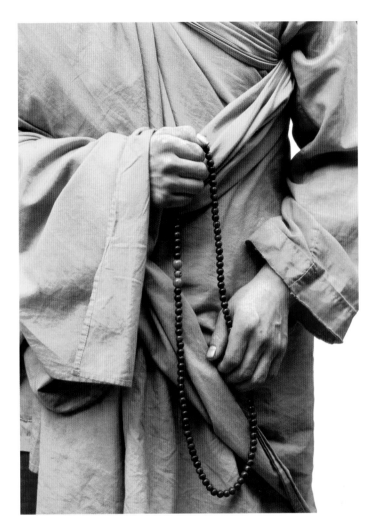

**right:** Buddhist monks in Tibet carry with them a circlet of 108 beads, a *mala*, to aid their invocating prayer.

## reciting holy words

As an alternative to the breath meditation, you can recite a meaningful or sacred word on each bead. Choose a word that resonates with you, maybe "peace" or "love." Christians might use an abbreviated version of the Jesus Prayer (page 158), repeating "Jesus" and "mercy" on alternate beads. Buddhists might prefer to chant "Om mani padme hum" each time (page 123). Work in the same way as for the breath meditation, but repeating with each out breath your chosen word or phrase out loud or silently. Each time, repeat your statement with intent, feeling its power fix its meaning and connotations in your mind. Since the divine name carries with it divine attributes, invoking it is thought to awaken the godlike essence within you.

## contemplation with a rosary

As well as using a string of beads to center yourself in the present, you can employ them for spiritual focus, as in the Roman Catholic tradition of meditating on the Mysteries—defining events in the life of Christ and the Virgin. In this tradition, the devotee contemplates three sets of five Mysteries while reciting the Hail Mary prayer on the five decades (rows of ten beads) of the rosary, depending on the day of the week or church calendar. These include the annunciation, crucifixion, and resurrection. If you have no religious background, try contemplating similar joyful, sorrowful, and glorious themes—love, humility, sacrifice, charity, repentance, hope—as you work through the beads on your secular prayer rope.

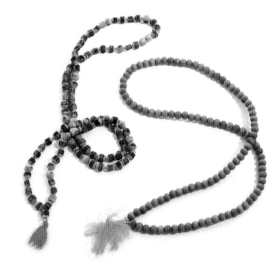

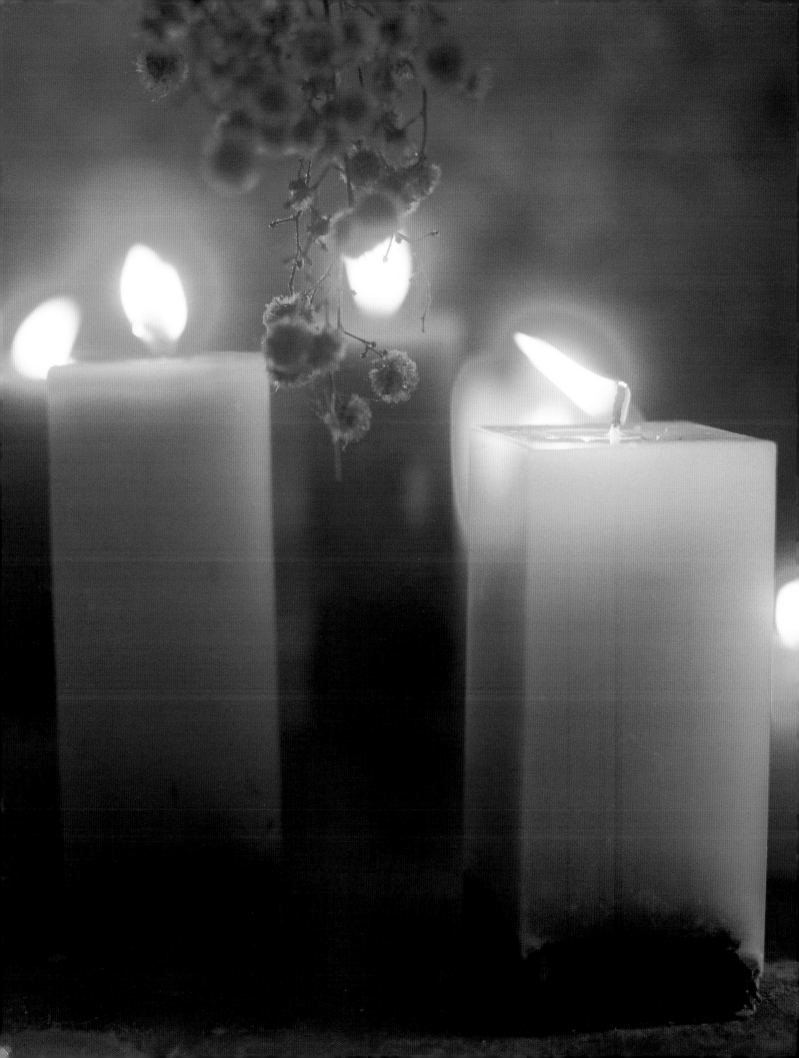

# meditation with a candle

The Trataka candle-gazing meditation uses the physical focus of a flame to help calm the mind. As you look only at the tip of the flame, your awareness of the flow of ideas through your brain slows down and eventually is effortlessly suspended. This type of "one-pointed," or single-focus, meditation can be particularly helpful at times of stress, when it can be difficult to keep your mind fixed on one thing. You will need a low table and a short candle.

❶ Sit comfortably upright on the floor, hands resting on knees or thighs (pages 22–27). Place the candle on a low table, level with your eyes.

❷ Settle yourself by watching your breath moving in and out for a moment, then focus your gaze on the tip of the flame, at the point at which its form and color disappear.

❸ Keep your gaze steady and uninterrupted on the flame for up to a minute, trying not to blink. Then close your eyes and visualize the flame in your mind's eye. Let it cleanse your mind, burning off thoughts and turning them into vapor.

❹ When the image has faded, open your eyes and repeat the gaze. As thoughts intrude, just let them burn away and return to the flame. Work for three minutes, using the image of the flame to cleanse your mind. Feel yourself becoming purer and more able to radiate your own light.

## concentration

Try not to focus on concentrating. Meditation should not be confused with concentration, which is simply a precursor to and step on the path toward meditation. Effort in concentrating creates more brain waves to interrupt the calm pond of the mind. When you feel yourself actively concentrating (you might notice frown lines on your forehead), switch your mind into an observing and witnessing mode, which erases traces of effort.

## i just can't be bothered

Meditation is rarely a straight path. Just as you seem to be getting somewhere, meditation becomes incredibly difficult and you lose the will, commitment, and momentum. After initial glimpses of what's possible, often you feel you're going nowhere. Keep starting over, harnessing the urge whenever it hits you. It may be connected with the change of the seasons, with new relationships and career changes, and with birth and death. Try setting less daunting targets: promise yourself to work with meditation for just a week or two. After the time period is up, look at what the practice has done for you and set yourself another target. Change methods: if just sitting loses appeal, take a meditation shower each morning, try walking with mindfulness, or sample a yoga class. Open yourself to every possibility, with the knowledge that when a method becomes a craving it's a distraction from meditation.

# focusing on a flower

Whether you select a perfect rose from the flower shop or work with a weed such as a daisy or dandelion plucked from the backyard, picking a flower can be the first step toward meditation. The focus of a single bloom not only entices your mind with sensual delight to remain in the present, it links you with the life of the natural world.

**❶** Sit or kneel comfortably upright (pages 22–25), holding the flower. Without slouching, bring the flower to eye level. Examine it using all your senses. Turn the bloom around and look at its form and color, savor its scent, however faint, brush the petals across your cheek, and think about how its constituent parts come together to create this unique form.

**❷** Close your eyes, steady and deepen your breathing, and try to conjure up the essence of the flower. Think not just of its tangible qualities, such as its physical form and scent, but also of its life force, its "flowerness."

**❸** Imagine yourself as the flower—a starting point might be to consider how many characteristics you share with the flower: its vulnerability, perhaps; its short period of blooming. When your mind wanders, constantly bring yourself back to the flower.

**❹** Now consider how at the molecular level you and the flower are composed of the same building blocks. Think about the fact that everything in the universe is made up of the same atoms. Go beyond this knowledge to merge yourself with the essence of the flower, and thus with the entire universe.

**❺** Work for three to five minutes, then come to gently. Keep the flower in a glass of water somewhere prominent in the home or on your office desk as a physical prompt to still the mind.

## mind-numbing methods

Use physical methods such as meditating on a flower or counting pebbles to engage with the act of meditation, but don't let them limit you. These tactile techniques have such enticing step-by-steps that you can get wound up in the mechanics, at which point you lose sight of the end point. Bear this in mind while you meditate and try not to get hung up on the method. Instead, liberate yourself by remaining open and looking beyond.

## the fabulous lotus

When you meditate on a lotus flower or adopt the yoga posture Padmasana, or Lotus Pose (page 23), for meditation, you merge with and embody one of Buddhism's most profound symbols. This plant grows with its roots in dank, murky water, yet takes nourishment from this detritus and rises out of it to flower in the air. This is seen as analogous to the art of meditation: although you are rooted in the real world with all its murky dealings and imperfections, you can transcend it through meditation to inhabit a world of peace, love, and light.

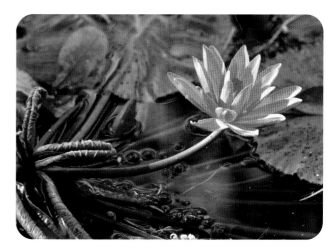

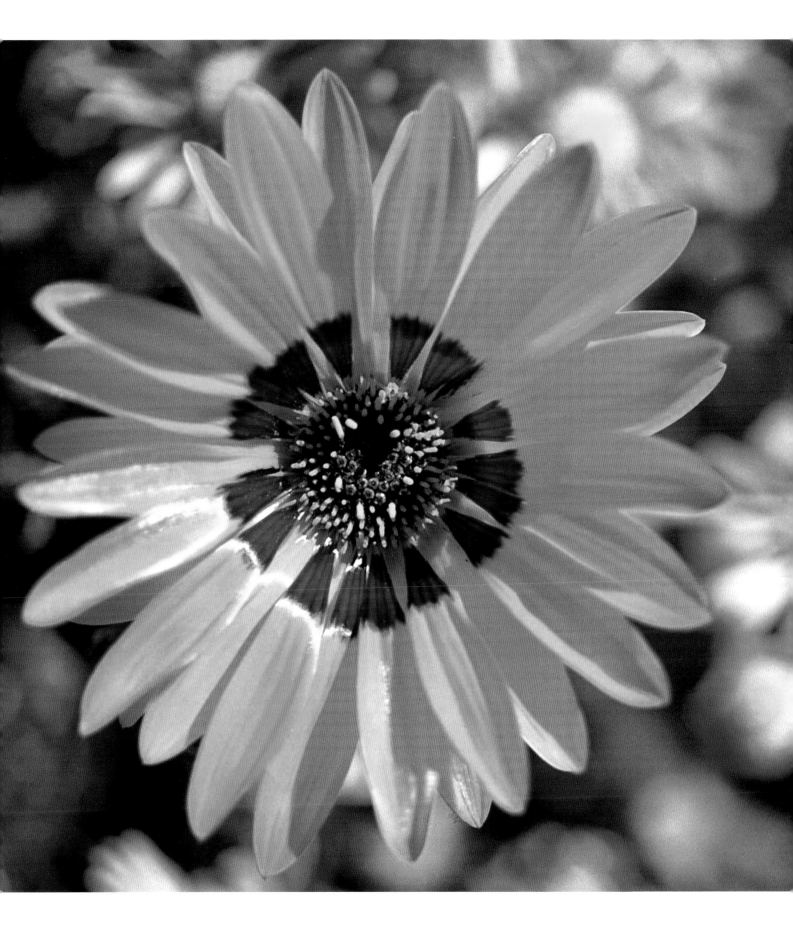

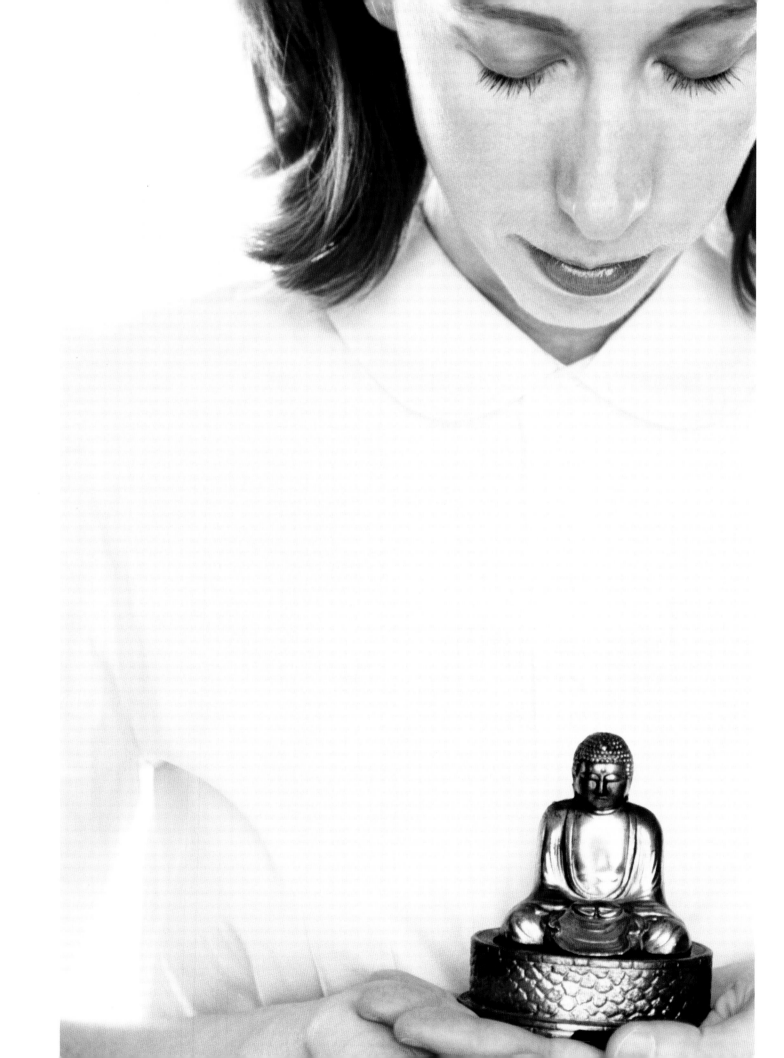

# meditating with a spiritual object

Some people find that starting to meditate comes more easily when the ritual is grounded in religious belief. Rather than meditating with a candle or flower, you might want the spotlight of a focused meditation to be on an object from your own religious background. Or perhaps images that have brought spiritual sustenance to people of faith the world over for centuries hold an appeal: an icon of the Virgin Mary, an image of Lord Krishna, or a statue of the Buddha. Bringing sole focus to an object so rich in symbolism does more than just still the mind and offer a retreat from the world, it can help your spirituality find its wings.

❶ Sit comfortably upright (pages 22–24) holding your object. Examine it to fix it in your memory in three dimensions, turning it around to view it from every angle. Pay particular attention to the facial expression and the energy of the eyes.

❷ Contemplate not only the physical form, but think about the virtues the statue embodies: perhaps compassion, love, serenity, or selflessness.

❸ Close your eyes and focus on your third eye, between your eyebrows. Visualize the image appearing in an intense light between and in front of your eyebrows. Focus your mind on its form and qualities; feel its essence with every sense. Every time your mind starts to drift, redirect it to the

object and allow it to glow brighter with each in breath. If the image does not appear when you close your eyes, open them and contemplate it again.

❹ Imagine divine energy flowing from your spiritual focus into your heart and let the qualities your image embodies merge with your inner self, building up inside you a reservoir of goodness and love for future use.

❺ Work for three minutes at first, extending the time you work with this form of meditation as you become more practiced. When you open your eyes and return to the outside world, feel divine energy glowing within and informing your every action and interaction.

## joining hands

The simple act of bringing the palms and fingers together in a universal symbol of prayer creates an instant entry point to meditation for every situation and any time of day.

**1** Sitting or kneeling with your spine erect (pages 22–25), bring your palms and fingers together in Namaskar Mudra (page 27), thumbs in front of your chest. Take a few moments to quiet your breath, feeling it lengthen and deepen.
**2** First meditate with eyes open, focusing on your joined hands. Think about two separate entities becoming one.
**3** Close your eyes and feel the contact between your palms, outside edge to outside edge, fingertips to wrists. With each in breath, feel love radiating in your heart; with each out breath, let this love flow into your palms. Join your hands and heart with an unending circle of energy. Work for up to three minutes before coming to.

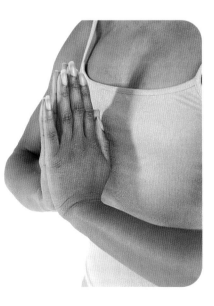

# mandala meditation

A mandala is a visual aid to meditation, a complex web of spiraling circles and interlinking squares representing the elements, directions, and energies at work in the universe. Contemplating its circular geometric design serves to focus the mind in the present while aligning you with these energies and revealing a pathway through complication and distraction to a still center. Mandalas range from huge, labyrinthine mazes that can be explored with the body to exquisitely intricate Tibetan *thankas* rendered on silk or in sand. The never-ending circle, symbol of the cyclical nature of life, is common to all forms. Many rituals surround the creation and contemplation of a traditional Tibetan mandala, but beginners might like to try these simplified exercises. Use the images on the next two pages or find one of your own.

❶ Sit or kneel comfortably upright (pages 22–25), with the mandala directly in front of you, propped up on a low table or pinned to the wall at eye level. Bring your focus to your breathing, watching it slow and deepen.

❷ Look at the mandala. Drink in its beauty, allowing it to speak to you without making judgments or forcing interpretations. Look at the range of options it presents to absorb the mind, and enjoy this feeling of plenty.

❸ Examine the corners and outer frame, letting them ground your mind and calm you. If thoughts intrude, acknowledge them and return to the colors and forms. In traditional Tibetan mandalas, the outer ring depicts flames that purify the person entering into meditation.

❹ Let your eyes be drawn in toward the center, following the paths you decipher. If you get lost or take turns that lead to a dead end, simply start again, appreciating the journey and not just the goal. Again, wipe away any intrusive thoughts as you pass along the visual trails. Meditating on these outer circles slowly prepares you to enter the inner sanctum of the central feature.

❺ Contemplate the heart of the mandala, often a central square known as the temple or palace. In a traditional mandala, the motif may be composed of lotus petals, representing the purity of the state of meditation you have achieved by passing through the mandala.

"Drawing makes me 100 percent happy. It's as good as the best food, exercise, or sex. As I work I get an immense sense of accomplishment; I feel complete, and everything else is irrelevant for a few seconds."

Georgia, artist

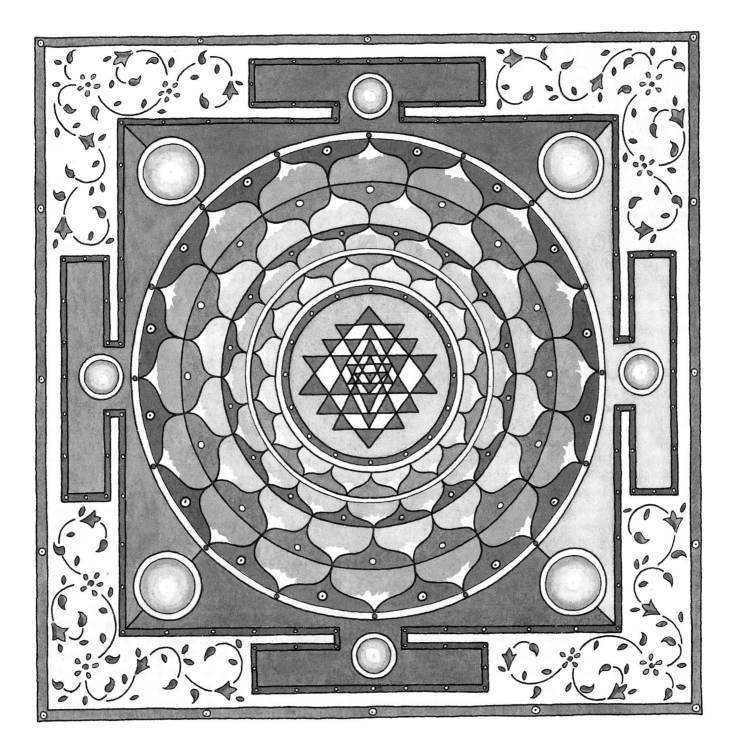

## creating a mandala

To make a mandala personal to you, start by drawing a circle (use a saucer or small plate) on a clean sheet of paper. In the center, mark out a square. Decorate the interior of the circle with concentric rings, using colors that attract you and employing intricate zigzag designs, snake motifs, and spirals. In the central square, draw or write something that has powerful significance for you—a sacred symbol or word, perhaps, or an affirmation to continue following your spiritual path. Be painstaking as you work, and focus on the task to the exclusion of everything else. Making the mandala is as much a contemplative act as meditating on it.

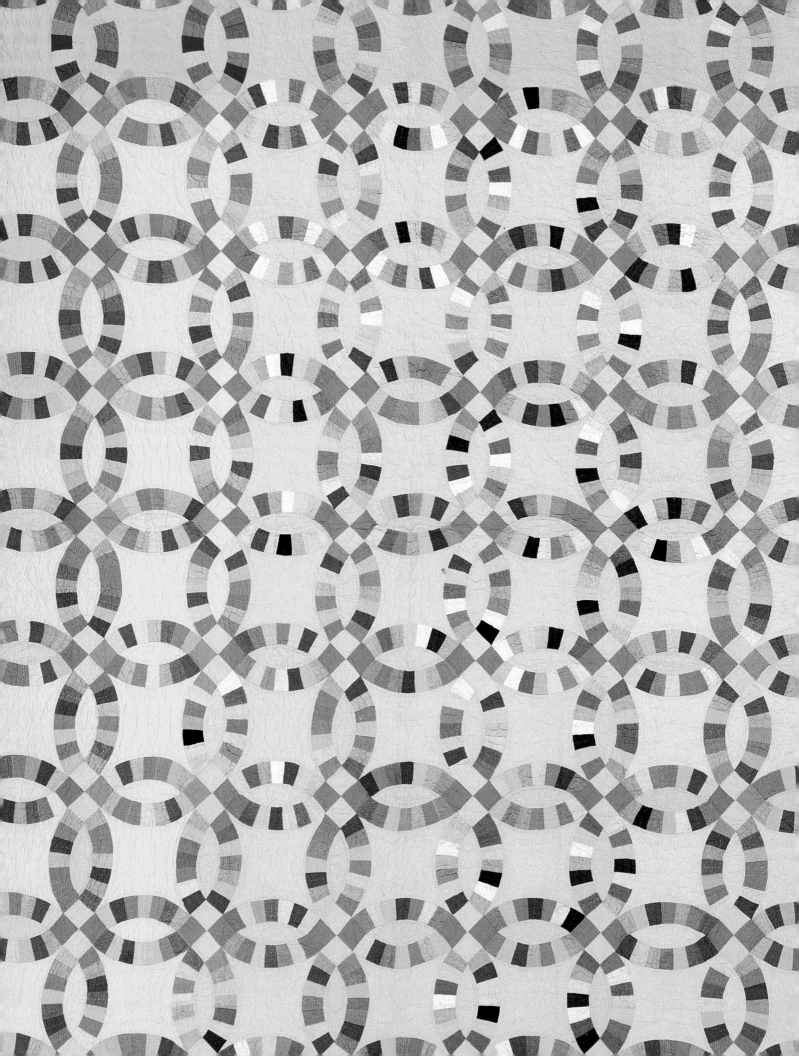

# contemplating celtic knotwork

If Eastern mandalas don't hit the spot for you, try contemplating Celtic knots. This has special appeal for those of us around the world with Irish, Scottish, Cornish, and Welsh family roots. A knot design is formed from a single thread that interlaces around itself without beginning or end. Like the circle of the mandala, as you follow it with your eyes your mind comes into communion with a pure, unending loop of continuity and connection. Celtic Christianity celebrates the interconnectedness of everything in the universe, and this gains ultimate expression in the knot motifs found since 800 B.C. adorning holy writings such as the *Book of Kells* and carved into ancient stone crosses. To use this complex geometric form for a mandala-style contemplation, look for a traditional knotwork motif.

❶ Sit or kneel comfortably upright (pages 22–25), with the image of the knot directly in front of you, propped up on a low table or pinned to the wall at eye level. Bring your focus to your breathing, allowing it to lengthen and deepen.

❷ Look at the knot design. Expand your mind to take in its wholeness and its lack of beginning or end.

## sacred geometry

Abstract geometric patterns created as a form of sacred expression are also key to Islamic art. In the medieval period, Islamic mathematicians computed theories of geometry that showed that all forms and shapes derive from the sphere. The whole and continuous nature of the circle connotes the infinite nature of the divinely created cosmos. It also alludes to the continual nature of daily devotion in the Muslim faith, with its five regular periods for prayer that are constant wherever one is on the revolving earth. You might like to contemplate an Islamic circular design, letting the hypnotic effect of the complex patterns, all based on degrees of a circle, give you insight into the macrocosm.

❸ Start to follow the thread. As it crosses over and under itself, let your eye and mind become fixed to the thread. Let this center you. If thoughts intrude, acknowledge them, but keep returning to the flow of the thread.

❹ Visualize in the circular winding the path of the sun in the sky and meditate on eternity. Think about the cyclical nature of the seasons and of life on earth: being born, living, dying, and returning to the elements.

❺ Ponder St. Augustine's words: "God is a circle, whose center is everywhere." Think also of the Zen notion that the act of sitting in meditation transcends time; the practice extends forever, from before time began endlessly into the future.

"As a child I enjoyed making patchwork; I started doing it again recently. I love the intense concentration on growing geometric designs, which have more meaning the bigger they get."

Lisa, computer technician

**left:** Detail of Double Wedding Ring quilt. This pattern of interlocking rings is a challenging piecing exercise and was particularly popular with quilters in America in the 1930s.

# zen puzzles

A koan is an unfathomable mental exercise or question pondered silently as a form of meditation in the Rinzai Zen tradition. The mind goes into overload with possibilities and impossibilities when faced with the insoluble nature of such puzzles, then starts to bypass received knowledge and the intellect and grasp the possibility of another, more unified, realm of connections. In considering koans you spring-clean the mind and adjust set patterns of perception and understanding. The result? A more intuitive way of responding to the world and an ability to adapt readily to new perspectives. Work with some of the suggestions here.

❶ Adopt an upright kneeling posture (page 25). If you prefer, wedge a cushion beneath your buttocks to take the strain. For extreme focus, tuck your toes under and sit on your heels so your weight compresses your toes. Keep the spine erect, ears and shoulders aligned, and look ahead.

❷ Place your hands in Cosmic Mudra (page 26). Half-close your eyes and focus ahead and just down, softening your gaze. Take your focus inside to watch your breath moving in and out effortlessly through your nostrils.

❸ When you feel calm, balanced, and in the present, start to consider the puzzle. Transcend the apparent paradoxes and open your mind to all possibilities. Give yourself the freedom to jump off at tangents; free your spontaneity, be intuitive, and enjoy the refreshment of new perspectives. Above all, cut away from worry.

❹ When it's time to finish, aim to keep the spaciousness of the open mind you experienced during the meditation by bypassing what stands for the intellect in everyday life.

## traditional koans

"What is the sound of one hand clapping?"
"What did your face look like before your parents met?"
"Bring me the sound of rain."
"Reveal the nature of the universe while washing up."

## alternative options

Ponder the Christian miracles—the Virgin birth, the resurrection—sensing the inability of the human mind to fathom divine understanding. Or look at the Sufi stories of Mullah Nasruddin, retold for centuries throughout the Middle East, which can be perceived simultaneously as moral tale, joke, and pointer along the spiritual path. For example: "One day Mullah Nasruddin went into a teahouse stating, 'The moon is more useful than the sun.' When asked why, he answered, 'We need more light at night than by day.'"

## looking for answers

Be warned that there are no set answers to koans, and to try to "solve" them is to lose their essence, which is to stir up and stretch the mind. Don't be tempted to analyze or interpret, just keep calling up the question. Don't close up alleys of thought by coming up with solutions. Just let the problem sit inside you, maturing over time.

**right:** The sudden illumination that comes from contemplating a paradox leads to spiritual realization.

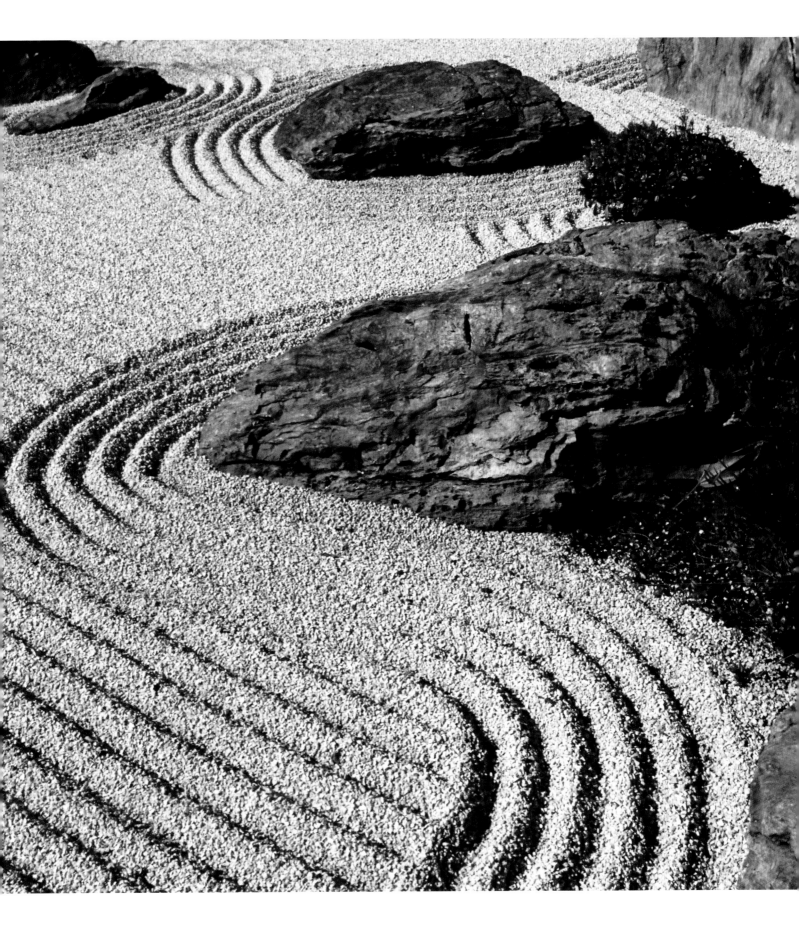

"Catch me the colors of a rainbow."

**Children's song**

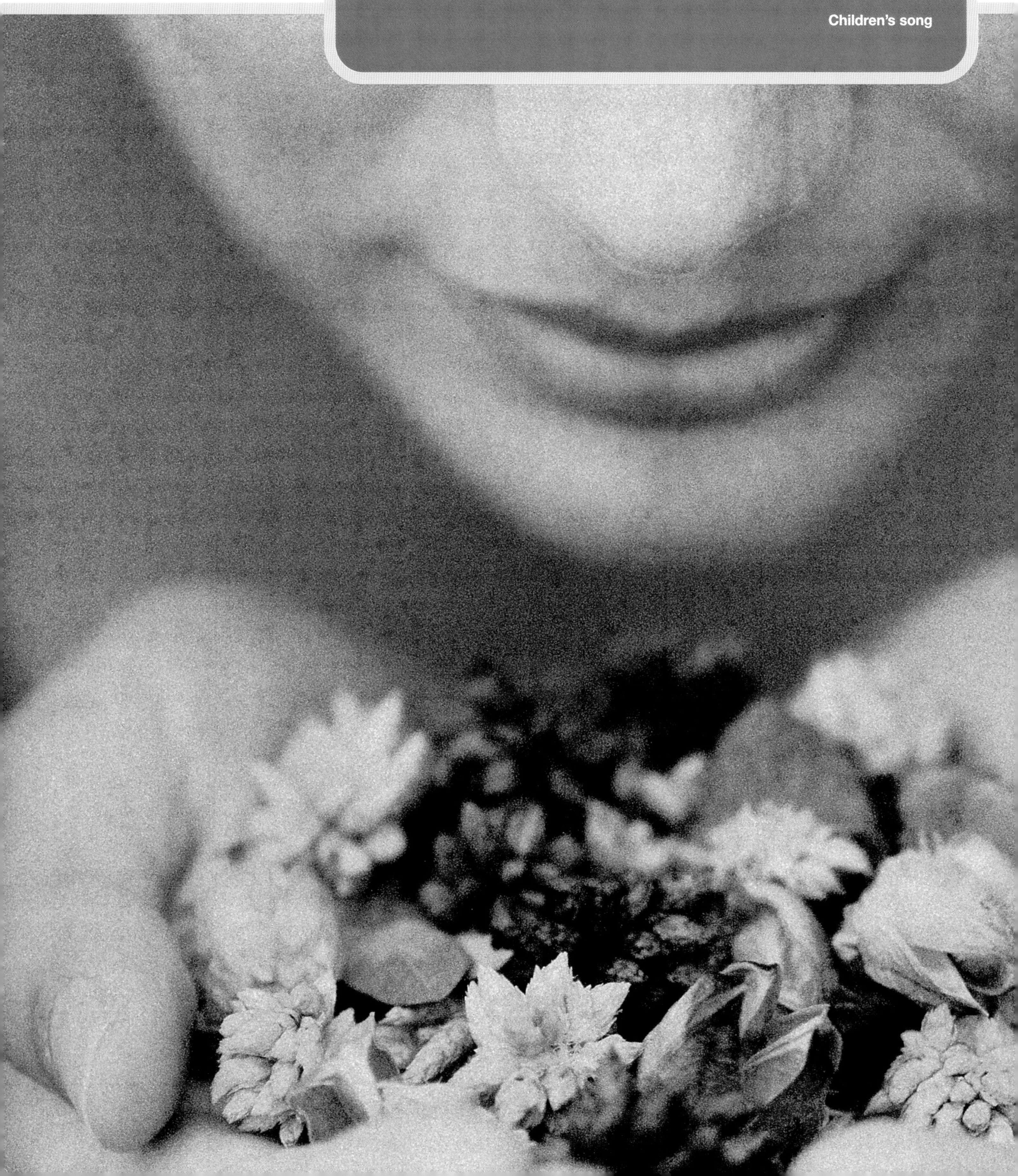

# sensory meditation

- **Sight meditation**
- **Touch meditation**
- **Smell meditation**
- **Incense meditation**
- **Taste meditation**
- **Sound meditation**
- **Music meditation**
- **Nature meditation**
- **Barefoot walking**
- **Sense withdrawal**

Sensations assault us all the time, and yet we tend to notice just the most pleasant or unpleasant. We need only pay attention to the messages the senses transmit to gain access to a vast world of awareness. Many forms of meditation work to switch on the senses, bringing alive sight, sound, and scent. Tempting touch and taste automatically brings us into instant contact with what's happening here and now and with the immediacy and amazing diversity of the big, wide world. Senses are powerful, primitive instincts that allow us to transcend intellect and the self-conscious "I" that filters everything we experience, separating us from the world. In a sound, a smell, a taste, we merge with the elements, opening up to the power and beauty of the universe while witnessing our habitual ways of framing perception and the paucity of this ego-centered interpretation. However, meditation is also about disengaging from the senses, discovering that we are not defined by sense perceptions, which are fleeting and ever-changing; each of us is more than what we see, hear, smell, touch, and taste. Being able to witness this ever-changing scenery from a still point takes us nearer to who we are: unchanging, settled, and in the now.

# sight meditation

Transform your perception of the world by learning to see everything afresh. Mindful attention to what's going on in front of your eyes expands your awareness. Find a special, quiet place to sit and watch the world (the view doesn't have to be spectacularly beautiful), or combine this exercise with the walking meditation ideas on pages 92–95.

❶ Sit or kneel in a comfortable upright position (pages 22–25) outdoors, hands resting on knees or thighs (pages 26–27). Center your head on top of your spine and keep your eyes alert. Calm yourself by focusing on the flow of breath in and out of your nostrils.

❷ Now stop thinking and start looking. Look at the scene in front of you as if for the first time. Note the real colors rather than the storybook hues we imagine the world to have (the sky isn't blue, grass is more than green, plowed fields are a rainbow of tones). Understand the sights as visual impressions without labels, like an impressionist painting.

❸ Bend forward and examine a blade of grass or stone up close. See how it blurs. Then look toward the horizon and try to decipher the specks. Point your chin to the sky and let its vastness widen your perspective. Without moving your shoulders, turn your head to look behind you, increasing the turn with every out breath.

❹ Imagine seeing the scene before you through the eyes of a baby or a dog. Then blur your senses by trying to imagine the sensations a flower perceives from this setting. Let your eyesight help free your mind from the impoverished nature of regular perception and alert you to the ways that you habitually frame your viewpoint.

## a living lens

Next time you go on vacation, leave behind your camera. Watch how, when faced with amazing events—whale-watching, reaching the summit of a hill, visiting an ancient monument—people habitually reach for the camera and see the event only through the camera lens. Experience the event in real time and fix it in your memory through your senses: feel it with your fingers, hear it, taste it. Let this be your lasting personal record.

## third eye meditation

Learn to see from more than one perspective. Adopt a sitting position and close your eyes. Without moving your eyes or frowning, focus your attention on the spot between your eyebrows (often referred to as the "third eye"). Turn your attention to your breathing, imagining the breath moving in and out through this spot. Feel it open to the world and endow you with a sense of expansion that helps you transcend your regular view of life.

## "Our eyes may see some uncleanness, but let not our mind see things that are not clean."

**Shinto prayer**

**right:** At the third eye, the body's three most important subtle energy channels meet and spiritual awakening develops. This painting of the White Tara shows her three eyes, which symbolize the purity of her body, speech, and mind.

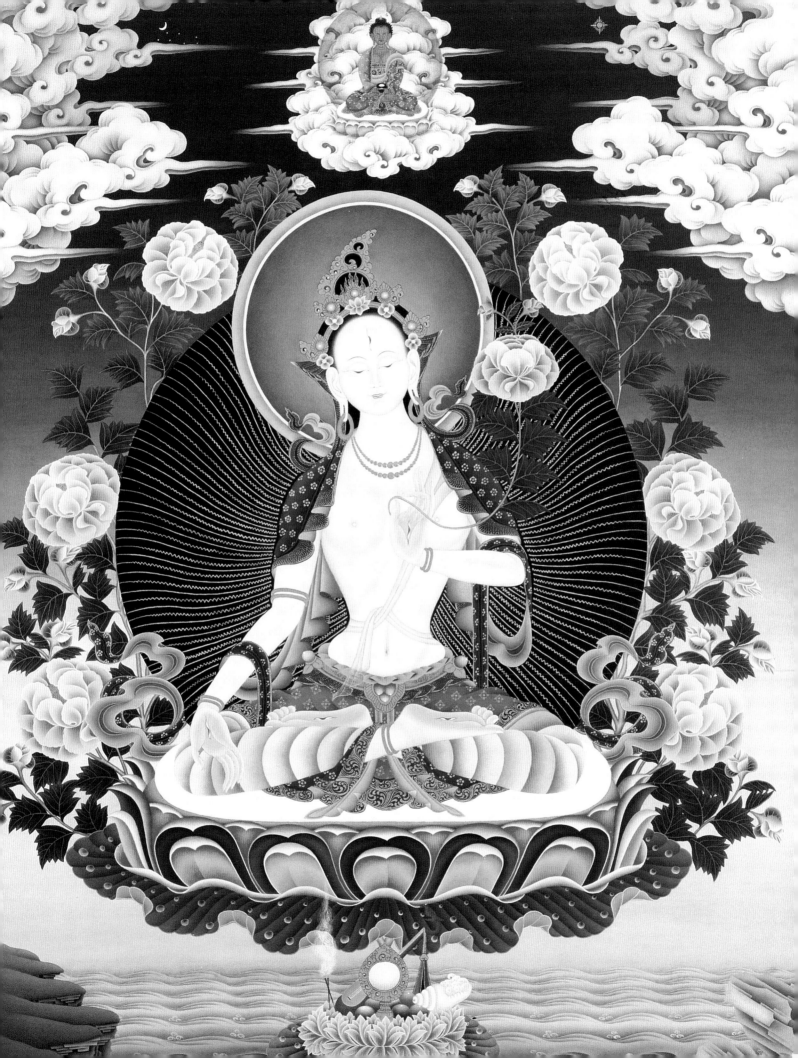

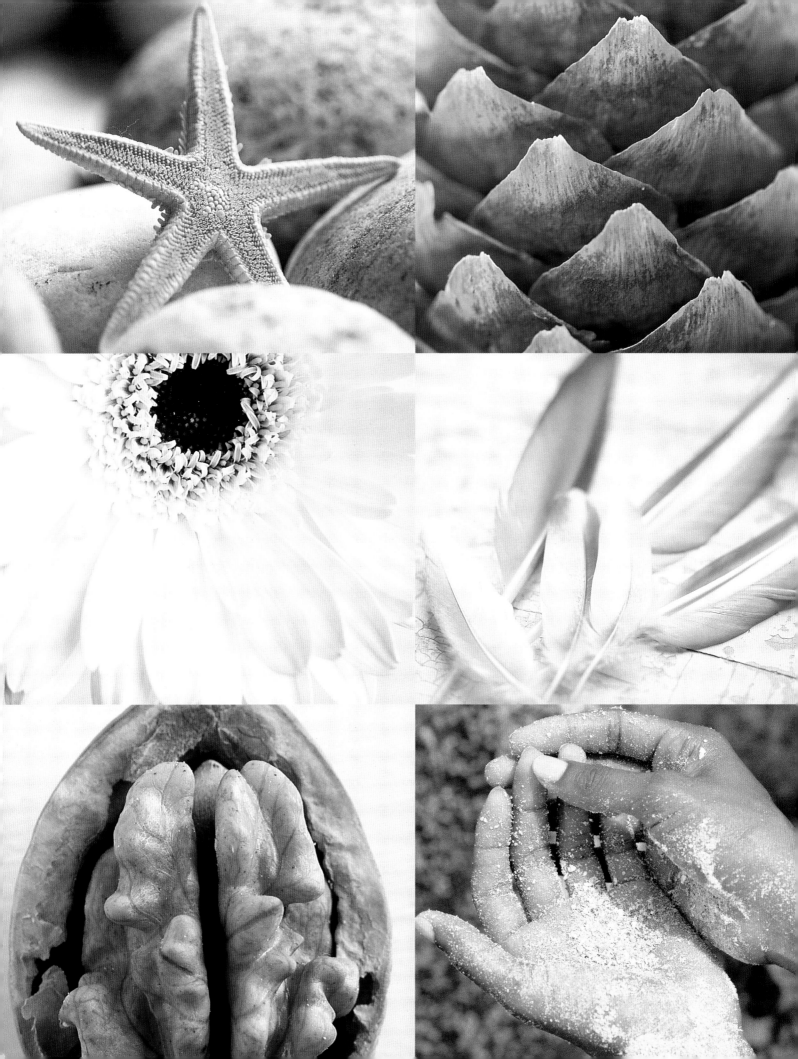

# touch meditation

Touch is the first sense that develops in the womb, and the body's largest organ, the skin, is exquisitely rich with nerve endings. Nevertheless, this sense is often the least explored. When we spend the day touching only computer keyboards and steering wheels, money and buttons on microwaves and phones, we deplete the spirit of sensory stimulation. Use this meditation to reacquaint yourself with the variety of tactile possibilities offered by the natural world. You will need to assemble a range of different-textured natural items. Good choices might include a feather and stone; oil, cornstarch, and water; rocks, clay or mud, and dry earth; driftwood and sheep's wool; and a dried leaf and a new bud.

❶ Assemble all the natural products in front of you. Sit comfortably upright on the floor (pages 22–23) and center yourself by turning inward to watch your breath moving in and out through your nostrils.

❷ In turn, pick up each object and devote thirty seconds to it. Roll it in your palm, run it through your fingers, brush it with your cheek and your lips. Pour yourself into the sensation and when other thoughts occur, simply acknowledge them and let them go before returning to the touch sensation.

❸ After five minutes or so, start to think about how much you shut out during everyday touch perception. Before finishing, vow to give more attention to touch sensations during the rest of the day.

## sensual touch

In a logical extension of touch meditation, take the techniques into the realm of lovemaking, one of the few everyday experiences that wake us fully to the present moment. Devote time simply to touching, steering clear of regular erogenous zones, and following wherever your creative energy leads. Start by resting your hands on your partner's body, letting them melt into the skin. Then touch with fingers and toes, lips and hair, and nuzzle with the nose. Take it in turns to caress and cuddle, stroke and lightly slap, tickle and twiddle, cup, stretch, and rub. Fan your palms over large expanses of skin and make figure eights and increasingly bigger circles. Inch your thumbs in a caterpillar crawl up the limbs and soles of the feet; knead and roll abundant flesh; rotate the knuckles in sensual massage. As you work, put your whole body into the strokes and bring your focus into the present, coordinating the strokes with the rhythm of your breath and remaining attentive to your partner's responses. Switching off to all but the nowness of sensation in this way expands the spirit as you both experience moments of openness and pure awareness.

> "Carving something really gentle and precise, I concentrate on the stone, aware only of what the chisel is doing."

**Simon, stonemason**

# smell meditation

The mind usually races between the senses without discrimination in a whirlwind of sensation. By bringing all your attention to one sense, you give the others a rest. In a sensory meditation, you also get to explore the world beyond your regular mental setup, expanding your repertoire of responses to people, places, and situations. Use this moving meditation to shed light on your habitual reactions and to help you begin to transcend them. You will need to be outdoors; being in the city or countryside makes no difference.

❶ Walk with your spine upright, your head balanced easily on top, your pace steady, and your gait relaxed. Bring your attention to your breath, coordinating your footsteps with your relaxed in and out breaths.

❷ When you feel centered and at ease, begin to notice the smells and scents of your surroundings. Start with the obvious: fast-food outlets and exhaust fumes, coffee shops and dry cleaners, grocery stores and flower stalls, fields of grass and farmyards, seaweed and salt water.

❸ Sample each sensation equally, like a wine taster, turning off your habitual responses and distinctions between pleasant and unpleasant and trying to savor each individual scent.

❹ Now try to discern less obvious olfactory sensations: puddles and shafts of sunlight, newspapers and leaves, hot metal and cold stone. Hone your appreciation of the scents as you try to focus on nothing but the essence of the smell, your awareness unfettered by your ego.

## games for children

Meditation games can be fun for children as young as two or three years old. Assemble a collection of scented objects from the garden and around the home. Choose the pleasant and the strange, the tear-inducing and the subtle, and try to include examples of floral and fruity scents as well as sweet and sour, stimulating and spicy, and cool and warm notes: you might include a bunch of lavender, vanilla pod, dried asafetida, a few drops of eucalyptus oil on a cotton ball, coffee grounds, a handful of cloves, milk, sliced lime, orange blossom, ground pepper, and fresh mint leaves. Ask children to sit in a circle and tie a scarf over their eyes, then pass them the scented objects, asking them to describe the smells. You'll be amazed by the descriptions, which aren't yet bound by safe, adult ways of responding. See if you can learn something from these fresh ways of perceiving stimuli.

"I love wearing a different perfume every day depending on my mood. Sometimes I feel like woody, spicy men's scents; when my head feels stuffy, I like light florals; and when I'm ready for some passion, I go for the really heavy Oriental-style blends."

Melissa, journalist

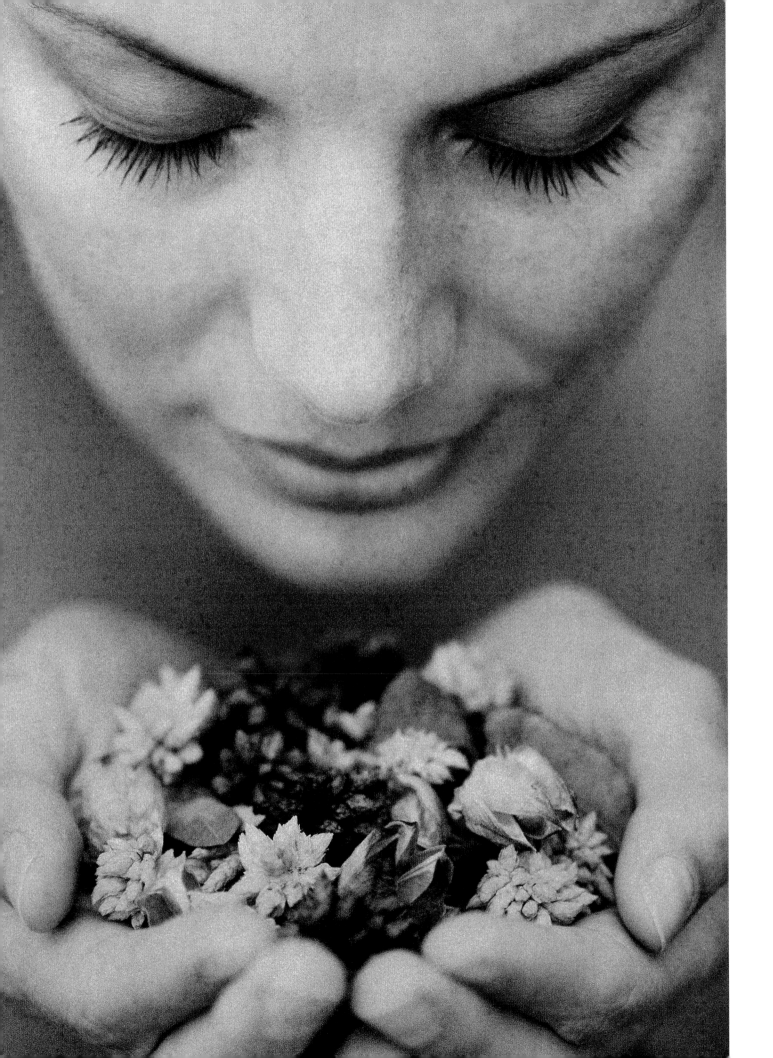

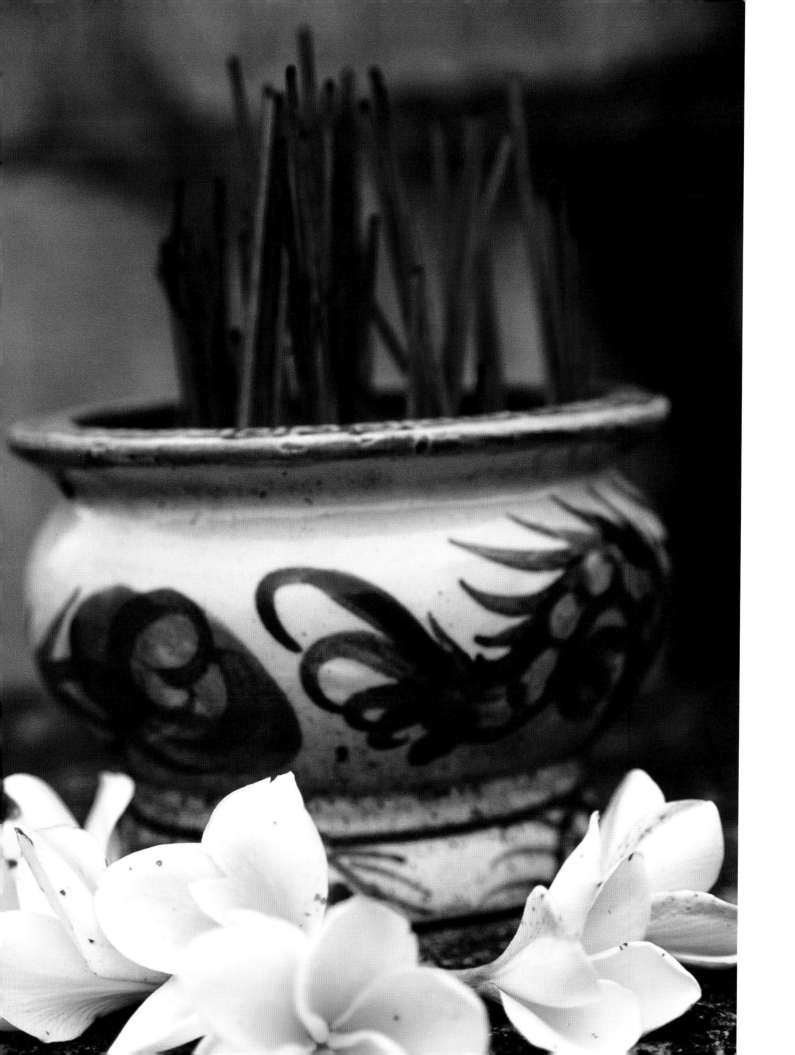

# incense meditation

In Japan, the art of making incense is more than highly skilled—it can be likened to a form of meditation that involves thirty years' study and much practice to master. Burning the resulting incense, *koh*, is also a meditation: one is urged to open up to the fragrance, to "listen" to the incense. The five key ingredients of traditional Japanese incense—aloe, clove, sandalwood, turmeric, and borneol—were set out in the Buddhist Sutras, or holy writings. The light scents of these recipes are said, among other virtues, to refresh and purify mind and body, bring alertness and peace to those with a hectic lifestyle, provide a companion in solitude, and even enhance communication with the divine. For this exercise you will need some traditional Japanese incense—as with fine wine, choose the best you can afford.

❶ Light the incense and place it in front of you, perhaps on a low table. Sit or kneel comfortably, with spine erect (pages 22–25), resting your hands on your knees or thighs (pages 26–27). Close your eyes.

❷ Take your gaze inside and watch your breath moving in and out. Let each in breath come naturally and feel the cool exhalation on the top of your upper lip.

❸ When you feel calm and grounded, begin to notice the scent of the incense. Let everything else drift away: when thoughts intrude, accept them without reacting and return again and again to the scent. Discern the top and base notes, the initial effect and the lasting impression; taste the scent on your palate.

❹ Open yourself to the scent; listen to what it has to say, however hard this might be at first. Keep switching off intellectual responses in favor of emotional and instinctive ways of intuiting.

❺ Before the incense burns away, offer up the exquisite scent in a spirit of openness and love for all to enjoy.

## cleansing the senses

In the Indian health-care tradition of Ayurveda, smoke inhalation is recommended to cleanse the senses and calm the mind. In the West, burning incense can be a good alternative. Choose sandalwood to soothe and rejuvenate frayed nerves; the scent is thought to deepen spirituality. Use frankincense to awaken. Its warm, balsamic scent boosts meditation by opening the mind and heart. Waft the smoke over your head as you pass, and use it to scent drying hair.

"I light incense when I get in from work. As it burns, it seems to clear all the day's troubles from my mind."

Yolanda, chemist

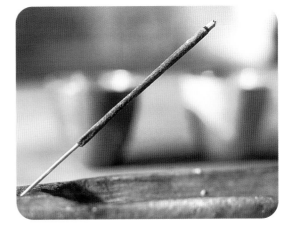

# taste meditation

These days, we tend to grab a processed fast-food meal and graze distracted and alone at a desk, in front of the TV, or on the move. We may not even be conscious of eating, or may miss meals because we are too busy to eat. In such a way, we lose a chance to nourish the spirit, relax the mind, and indulge the senses while refueling the body. We also deprive ourselves of an everyday way of experiencing the truth of the Sanskrit aphorism, "Thou art that." We are what we eat, so use this eating meditation to awaken your awareness and remind yourself of the joy of nourishing mind as well as body.

❶ Before you eat, make sure you really are hungry. Then, at every meal or snack, sit down to eat at a table, with others if possible.

❷ Remove all distractions and turn off the television or radio. Sitting upright (a great aid to digestion), bring yourself into the present and center yourself by noticing your smooth, even breathing and letting go of raised emotions.

❸ Take your attention to your plate. Look at the food before you as if seeing it for the very first time. Note its colors, temperature, textures, and arousing blend of aromas. When other thoughts pass through your mind, let them pass, constantly bringing yourself back to the reality of the food.

❹ As you handle the food, sense the textures: smooth and rough, tough and tender, oozing and sloppy.

❺ Close your eyes as you place a morsel in your mouth. Pause before chewing and let the flavors activate the taste buds at various points on your tongue. Let the taste sensations fill your consciousness.

❻ As you chew, feel the muscles in your jaw and neck become involved, sense the connections between hand and brain as you lift your fork, and feel your teeth coming together. Slow down to appreciate each mouthful in the moment; throughout the meal, keep coming back to this.

❼ After finishing, simply sit still in silence for a few minutes. Take your attention to your body: visualize the food circulating through your body's systems and being transformed into energy.

## food connections

Eating connects us not just to the raw ingredients of the foods as we swallow and digest them, miraculous as this is, but also to all those people who made it possible for the food to reach the plate. As you eat, ponder those connections: think of the farmers who tilled the land, the truck drivers who brought the food across the country, the men and women who created the raw materials for your stove, the engineers who designed the gas supply line that enables you to cook. Eating brings each of us into an intimate connection with people we will never meet and times that have passed. Let this interdependence expand your view of your place in the world and allow you to appreciate the shared nature of the simplest everyday tasks.

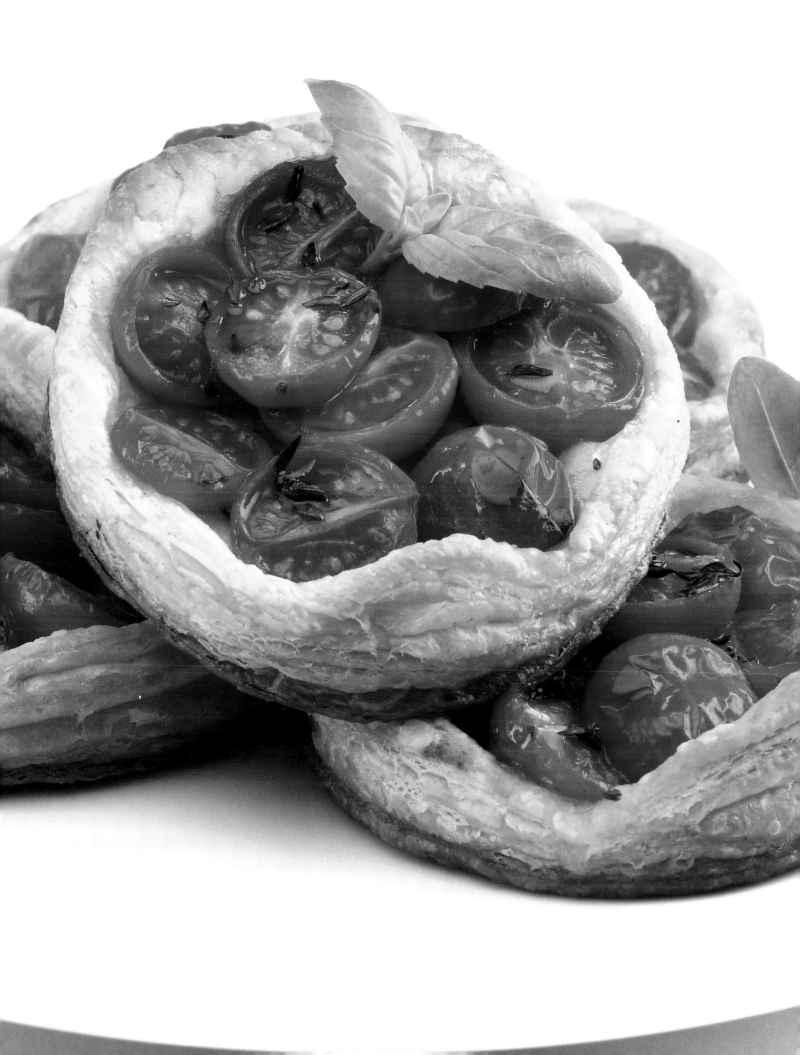

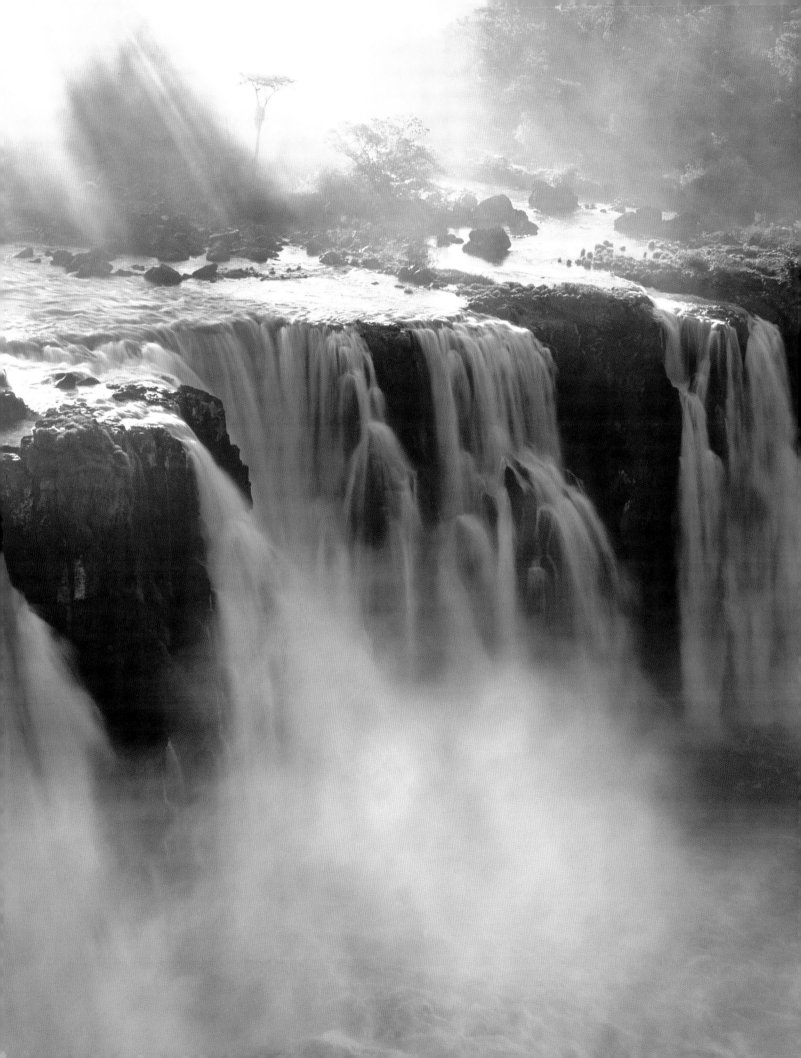

# sound meditation

Sharpen your hearing with the following meditation, which allows you, in the midst of everyday life, to tune in to the humming of the globe. Despite being surrounded by a deafening audio landscape, we are often aware only of those sounds we want to hear. This exercise teaches you how to open up to every type of sound, suspending judgment and widening perceptions. The composer John Cage worked with the belief that every sound is a viable source for composition. Gain your own sonic liberation with this meditation.

❶ Wherever you are right now, stop what you're doing. Stand or sit up straight and shut down all your senses but your hearing. Close your eyes if this helps.

❷ Focus on the sounds immediately around you. What can you hear with your left ear? What sounds can you catch with your right? What can you hear in front of and behind you?

❸ Now listen outside your immediate surroundings. What can you hear behind you? What sounds are in the building? What can you hear outdoors? Don't just focus on pleasant sounds; adjust your perception to appreciate the blaring siren, the shriek of a car alarm, a shout, and a whining child. Don't label the sounds, just appreciate their tone and timbre. Try to extend your hearing beyond the traffic, birdsongs, wind, and rustling of trees to the inaudible and sense the universe humming.

## inner sound

When you have practiced the listening meditation for some time, start to take your raised perception of sound inside you. Ancient sages in India taught that within each of us is the sound of the universe vibrating—shabda. After sitting in meditation with eyes closed for some time, or during the yoga posture Savasana (pages 28–29), when you feel calm, centered, and at peace, start to listen within. It may be helpful to block your ears at first and to focus on the third eye area between the eyebrows. Sense a ringing, humming, or deeper rumbling. Tune into the sound, following where it leads; it may help to take your focus to your solar plexus, the site of the navel chakra (pages 120–21). Do nothing but pay attention to the sound; when your mind wanders, simply pin it back to the sound vibration.

## focusing meditation with sound

Use sound to mark the boundaries of a meditation session. Some people like to chime finger cymbals or ring a bell to cleanse the energy of the meditation space before starting to practice and after finishing. During meditation itself, you might like to use a pair of Chinese meditation balls to focus your sense of hearing and draw you into the present. Cup the balls in the flat of your palm and gently circle to create a constant ringing. This practice also calls in your sense of touch.

# music meditation

Herbie Hancock—jazz musician and Buddhist—describes jazz as "a music of the moment." Improvisation allows him to capture the essence of the present and express it; to provide for listeners an unmediated glimpse of the realm of the infinite. Twentieth-century minimalist classical composers aim through unceasing repetition and reduction to create what Phillip Glass called "intentionless music" that avoids recollection and anticipation and challenges our perception of time by using imperceptible changes to keep listeners and players in the present. Both types of music lend themselves well to this listening meditation. You will need a CD, cassette, or record player with a remote control.

❶ Sit between and in front of the two speakers in a comfortable upright pose (pages 22–24), hands resting on thighs or knees (pages 26–27). Close your eyes and listen to nothing but the movement of your breath in and out for a few minutes.

❷ When you feel centered and solidly rooted to the ground, start the music with the remote control. Switch off your habitual reactions and let yourself be drawn in by the mood of the music—the combinations of instruments, the themes stated and restated, the pattern of changes, the process gradually unraveling. Allow time to be suspended.

❸ Start to follow the voice of one particular instrument; it doesn't have to be the main melody line. Let it take you where it goes. When thoughts intrude, swat them away and return to the sounds.

❹ Become aware of the musicians playing: hear wind players grabbing breaths; note the squeaks of fingers on keyboards and guitars. Then sense the intention of the composer slowly unfolding. When the piece comes to an end, sit in silence for a few minutes, savoring how it felt to be lost in music.

## mindful playing

When playing an instrument, try to release yourself from technique, from the mechanics of "playing well." As a form of meditation, take your focus to the instrument's tone and try to fuse yourself with its sound as you play. In Suizen, a blowing meditation from the Zen tradition, you aim to transcend the mere playing of correct notes to become the sound and that which it represents—often drawn from nature. Visualization can help—imagining yourself as the theme of the piece, perhaps the sea or a bird. Musicians learning Indian ragas are taught that by listening with focus to the music while playing, the raga releases its presiding spirit and the player merges with it.

## meditation vibes

Use these pieces as a springboard for your own selections, looking in the library or browsing through the classical and jazz sections of good music stores.

"Impressions" from *Impressions* by John Coltrane

"Modal" from *Abstract* by the Joe Harriott Quintet

"Nothing Without You" from *Mustt Mustt* by Nusrat Fateh Ali Khan

*In Concert 1972* by Ravi Shankar and Ali Akbar Khan

*Music from the Morning of the World* by The Balinese Gamelan

*Cantus in Memory of Benjamin Britten* by Arvo Pärt

*Discreet Music* by Brian Eno

*Variations for Wind, Strings, and Keyboards* by Steve Reich

*Jesus' Blood Never Failed Me Yet* by Gavin Bryars

*Selected Ambient Works, Vol. I* by Aphex Twin

"It's like food. Sometimes I feel like I haven't eaten for days and just have to listen to music."

Stephen, photographer

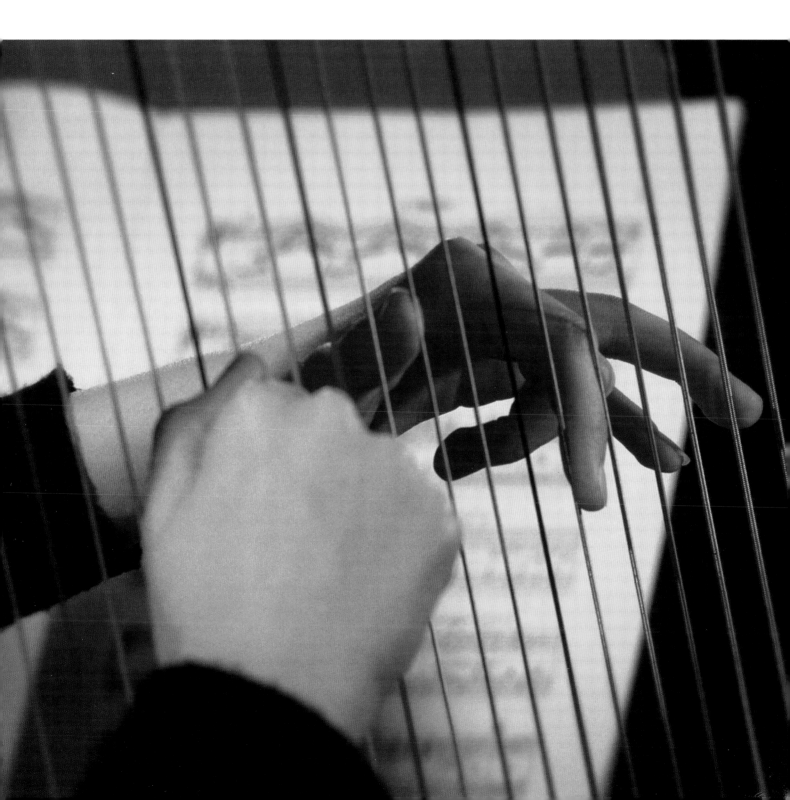

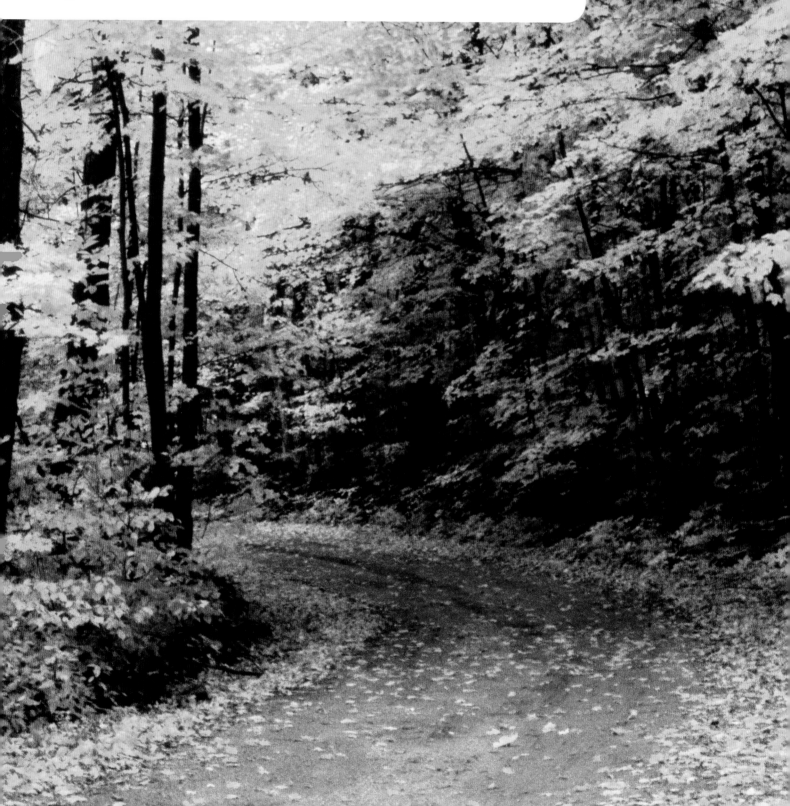

"When I paddle out to sea, waiting for the wave and just watching the backs of the waves, I feel tiny and insignificant in the universe."

Garry, canoeist

# nature meditation

This fresh-air meditation has the power to lift a bad mood and shift "stuck" thoughts. It also aims to help you find the connection between the human spirit and the natural world, to experience the understanding that we are composed of the same molecules and atoms as rocks, rivers, plants, and birds. You don't have to leave the city to connect with nature: it's there all the time in the wind and rain, falling leaves and the self-seeded weed that breaks through a crack in the sidewalk.

❶ Go for a walk outdoors. Walk briskly for a few minutes to rid your mind and senses of stale impressions from previous activities. Take a few deep breaths and exhale all your mental worries and physical aches and pains.

❷ Let your pace settle into the rhythm of your breathing, allowing the in breath to come naturally.

❸ Start to notice the world around you. Look down at the earth and up at the sky. Feel the temperature of the air and look for clues to the season.

❹ Now start to slow your pace, making it more deliberate. Quiet your mind and heart; as thoughts come, note them, then let them pass, until you find yourself doing nothing but moving in nature.

❺ Try to see, hear, and experience the natural world without labels: see birdsongs, smell the sky, feel the horizon. Then connect the exterior with your interior: contemplate how you have inside you the same water, minerals, and heat. Transcend the differences. Work for a total of five minutes.

## bringing the natural world inside

Bring the elements of the natural world indoors, reserving space at your altar (pages 20–21) for fire (incense or a candle), water (a bowl of water), earth (a crystal or a pot of a spiritually uplifting herb such as holy basil), and air (hang a wind chime by an open window). Connect with them before starting to meditate.

## exercising outdoors

Whenever possible, practice your yoga, tai chi, or qi gong routines outside. There's no better way to experience the spacious feeling of being part of the greater scheme of things than to hold a pose while gazing into the blueness of a summer sky. The sensations intensify when practicing in the dark, when the sparkle of stars sets the earth in the bigger picture of the cosmos.

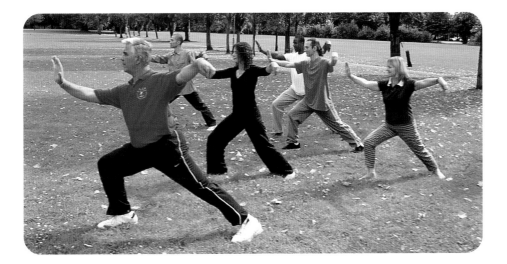

# barefoot walking

The feet contain a wealth of nerve endings and pressure sensors, connecting them with every part of the body. When these remain unchallenged by wearing shoes and walking on flat, even surfaces, body and mind become numbed. This barefoot walking meditation is based on the Japanese tradition of *takefumi*, walking on bamboo, as espoused by Samurai warriors, who equated the feet with the soul. It challenges the feet with unexpected combinations of textures that enliven the body, awaken the senses, and encourage the mind to open to new possibilities. You will need to set aside some space outdoors.

❶ Prepare a walking meditation pathway by assembling in a row trays of different-textured objects for the feet to encounter. Good examples include gravel and pebbles of varying sizes; grass, sand, and mud; bowls of very warm and ice-cold water; lengths of bamboo cut in half, rounded side up; and broom handles.

❷ Stand at the beginning of the pathway and center yourself by standing upright, your body weight balanced between both feet, spine straight, and the crown of your head pulling toward the sky. Watch your breath moving in and out for a few minutes.

❸ Start walking along the pathway. Carefully ease your body weight onto each surface, paying attention to new sensations and watching how different parts of the foot react to different surfaces. Experiment by shifting your body weight from side to side and forward and back.

❹ When you tire of one sensation, move to the next station on the pathway. While taking your full awareness to the sensation in your feet, notice also how the rest of your body responds to the changing stimuli. If something feels too painful, breathe into that area of the foot, trying to bear the pain for slightly longer than you think possible, then move to the next station.

❺ When thoughts intrude, breathe them away and return to the sensations you can feel in your feet. Work for five to ten minutes once a week.

## grounding the body

Before or after the barefoot meditation, use this grounding yoga exercise to connect the soles of the feet to the ground. Stand with feet hip-width apart, parallel on the outer edge (pigeon-toed). Distribute your weight equally between both feet, and on each foot feel the base of the big and little toes and both sides of the heel pressing down. Extend your body weight up from these points. Lift your toes, splay them, hold, then set them back on the floor one by one, trying to maintain a gap between each toe. Feel your toes and the four parts of each foot anchored to the floor, imagining when you breathe that the in breath starts six feet beneath the surface, and that with each exhalation you send nervous tension down into the ground. To check your solidity, sway forward and back and from side to side until you find a point just forward from your heels at which you gain an effortless energy lift.

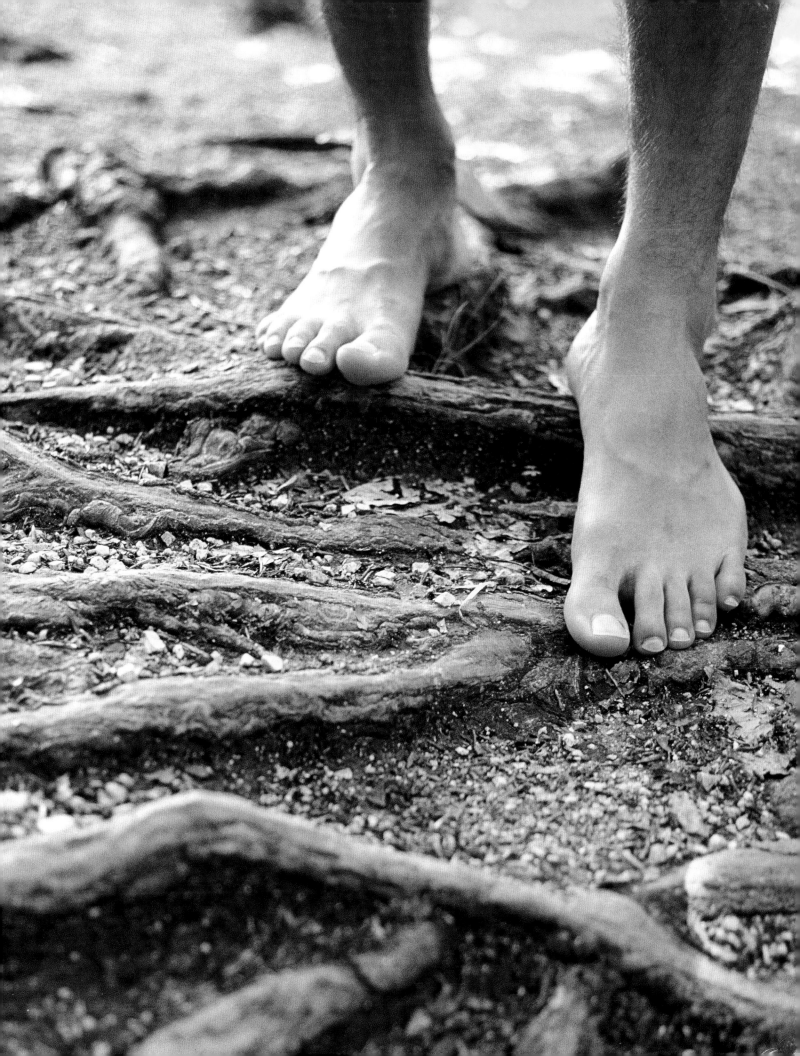

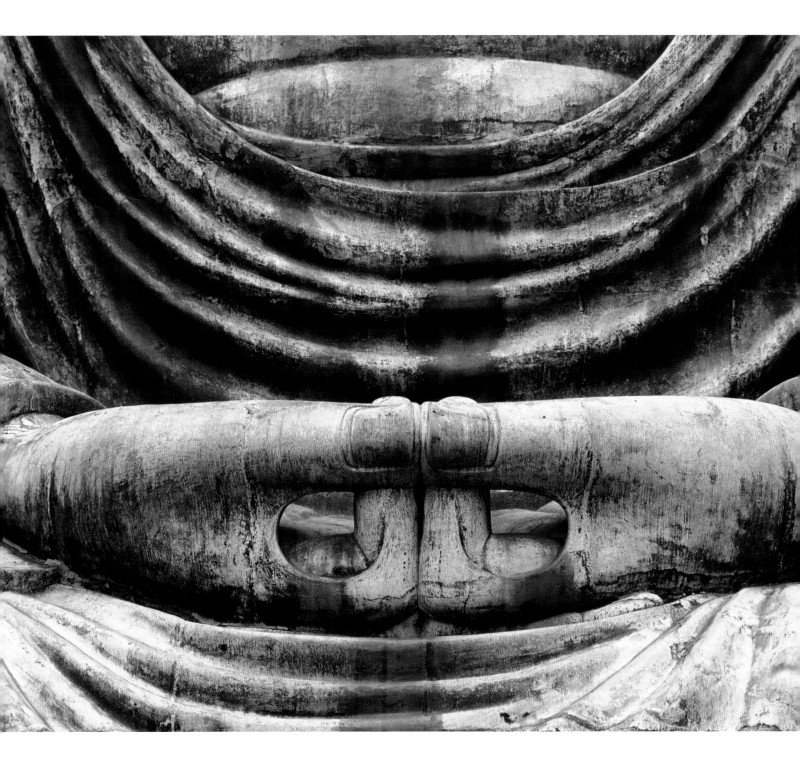

"It's such a relief just to stop working and be completely relaxed for once."

Kim, medical student

# sense withdrawal

Some traditions teach that sense meditations are useful only to a point. Yes, they reduce the avalanche of sensations to a manageable level, allowing us to experience each one fully. But they may become a trap, distracting from the ultimate aim of finding the real you, which is unchanging amid the ever-fluctuating world of impressions. The English Roman Catholic Cardinal Archbishop Basil Hume spoke of how the senses allow us only temporary "shafts" of experience of ultimate reality, according to their limited abilities. The aim of the spiritual seeker should be to transcend these deficient sources with the mind to experience, unfiltered, the pure glory of creation in the now. Let this sense-withdrawal meditation direct you along this path.

❶ As you go through your day, bring your attention to each of your senses. When you see something remarkable, appreciate it, but remember that your sight constantly receives new impressions, which are temporary, unlike the real you inside.

❷ When you notice a sound, enjoy it, then reflect on the ever-moving nature of the soundscape and compare this to the solidity of the you witnessing it.

❸ Appreciate every tactile sensation in the gym, at the dinner table, and in bed with a lover, but try to retain an awareness of the immutable, steadfast nature of the self inside that witnesses this fleeting world of sensation.

# yoga sense withdrawal

❶ Sit upright (pages 22–24), with the hands in Cosmic Mudra (page 26). Draw up and out of the pelvis equally on both sides from hip to armpit. Tuck your chin toward your throat and extend through the back of the head. Close your eyes and focus on the out breath, allowing it to lengthen from the abdomen up. Let the in breath come easily.

❷ Start to bring your senses inward. Withdraw your sight from your eyes and look within. Bring your hearing in from the ears to listen within the body. As you inhale, take your sense of smell inside from the nostrils. Let your sense of taste be absorbed from the tongue. Withdraw your sense of touch from the fingers and hands and from the skin itself.

❸ Reside within, simply watching your breathing, losing all thoughts and experiencing stillness. Watch thoughts pass through your brain with disinterest. You may feel a sense of merging, of not knowing where your body ends and where the outside world starts.

❹ After finishing the meditation, sit in silence for a while, becoming attuned to the outer world, but retaining within yourself an inner awareness of completeness.

**left:** Only in contemplating sacred emptiness does the Buddhist find salvation from the vain emptiness of the world.

"The body must be as transparent as air."

**Li Tao Tze**

# active meditation

- Meditating with yoga
- Making prostrations
- Whirling meditation
- Qi gong sequence
- Walking with mindfulness
- Just walking
- Gardening with mindfulness
- The art of calligraphy
- Shower power
- Clutter clearing
- Cleaning meditation
- Conscious cooking
- Baking bread

If you're the kind of person who likes to be active, you may find it easier to start meditating with movement exercises. This form of meditation also suits people who tend to overintellectualize. It holds appeal for those with busy lives, since you don't need to set aside a separate time for practice. The active meditations that follow also make a good warm-up for sitting meditations. When performing a yoga sequence or taking a walk, many people find the mind calms readily, lulled by the rhythm of motion. Energy patterns also settle into harmony. The aim of yoga and qi gong is to treat every posture as a meditation. In a yoga pose, your mind is anchored in the present as it goes out to hands and feet, legs and arms, moving in diverse directions. The novel ways of seeing in each posture—eyes fixed to the knees one moment, the sky the next—disorient you from everyday ways of being. In qi gong, you take on a state of mind that connects you to everything, understanding that the world is inside you as you are within it. Then, even while moving, you experience calm. Taoism teaches that stillness in stillness is not real stillness; only when there is stillness in the midst of movement does the nature of the universe reveal itself.

# meditating with yoga

Surya Namaskar, the Sun Salutation, is a continual series of movements coordinated with the breath that, when practiced at sunrise and sunset in a flowing sequence, brings body and mind into balance with the natural world. Work on each movement separately first to fix it in your memory, then practice moving slowly through the sequence. Do not hurry this learning process or worry too much about the breathing. Add the breathing instructions when you start to speed up, building up to fourteen repetitions of the sequence, seven on each side. Soon you will find yourself moving in meditation: the stretching of the limbs, the smooth in and out breaths, and the constant thought of the sun become your focus, wiping out all other thoughts and sensations. You become a pure expression of the movement of the sun across the sky. Try to work outside when possible, and start facing east, the point on the compass where the sun rises every day.

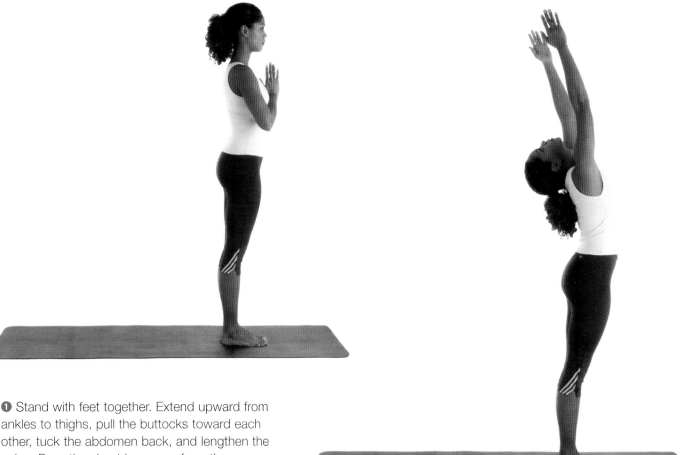

❶ Stand with feet together. Extend upward from ankles to thighs, pull the buttocks toward each other, tuck the abdomen back, and lengthen the spine. Drop the shoulders away from the ears and extend up the back of your neck, as if suspended by a thread from the crown of the head. When you feel calm and stable, bring your palms into Namaskar Mudra, the prayer position, in front of your chest (page 27). Look forward and visualize the sun.

❷ With an inhalation, extend your arms overhead, shoulders relaxed, arms covering the ears. Then stretch backward, arms apart, and look behind. Absorb the sun into your opened chest.

❸ Exhaling, bend forward from the hips, legs straight if possible, planting your palms on either side of your feet and relaxing your head between your arms. Don't worry if you have to bend the knees: work on straightening them as you exhale. Let the sun's rays warm your lower back.

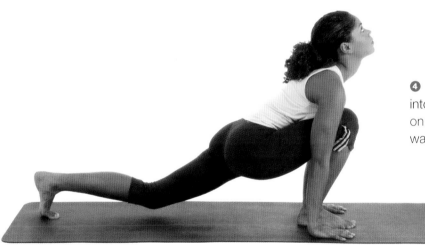

❹ On the next inhalation, take the left leg back into a lunge position, right heel remaining flat on the floor. Look up, raising your chest to the warming sun.

❺ Take the right leg back and hold yourself on hands and feet like an angled plank in a push-up position, looking slightly forward. Keep the hips raised. Feel the sun on the length of your spine.

# "Yoga keeps me centered when everything's going crazy at home and work."

**Nicoletta, interpreter**

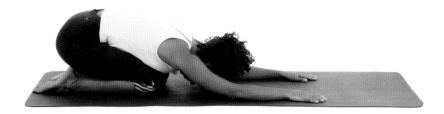

**❻** Exhaling, relax back onto bent knees (heels and toes touching), arms forward and palms still rooted to the spot.

**❼** On an inhalation, press forward on your arms, buttocks in the air, then press on your hands to bring the chest up, dropping the head back. Tuck your elbows into your waist. Relax your shoulders and try not to compress the lower back.

**❽** With the next exhalation, push your hips toward the sky, extend out of the shoulders, and work to press the heels down. Absorb the sun into the top of your back and shoulders.

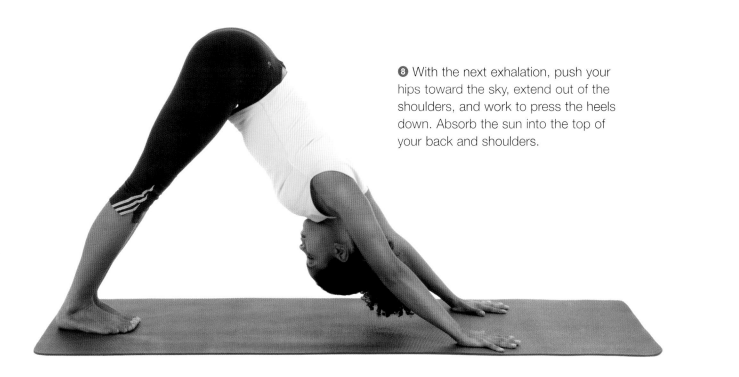

**9** Step your left leg forward with an inhalation back into the lunge pose and look up again, as in step 4.

**10** Bring your right leg forward with an exhalation and push your tailbone to the sky, working to straighten the knees, as in step 3.

**11** Draw your hands into prayer position up your body and overhead with an inhalation. Open your arms and extend backward, as in step 2.

**12** Bring your hands back into prayer position in front of your chest with the exhalation, bowing your head to the sun. Repeat all the steps, this time working with the opposite leg.

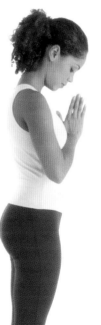

# making prostrations

Lying fully prone from forehead to toes, body flattened on the ground, is a profoundly humbling and calming pose of self-surrender. As the ultimate from of supplication, it takes on spiritual significance in many religions, part of the salat prayer ritual of millions of Muslims five times a day and repeated by Greek Orthodox monks reciting the Jesus Prayer (page 158). This exercise is adapted from the Buddhist tradition; even if you have no religious background, try the deep and reverent stance to help rein in an inflated ego before starting to meditate.

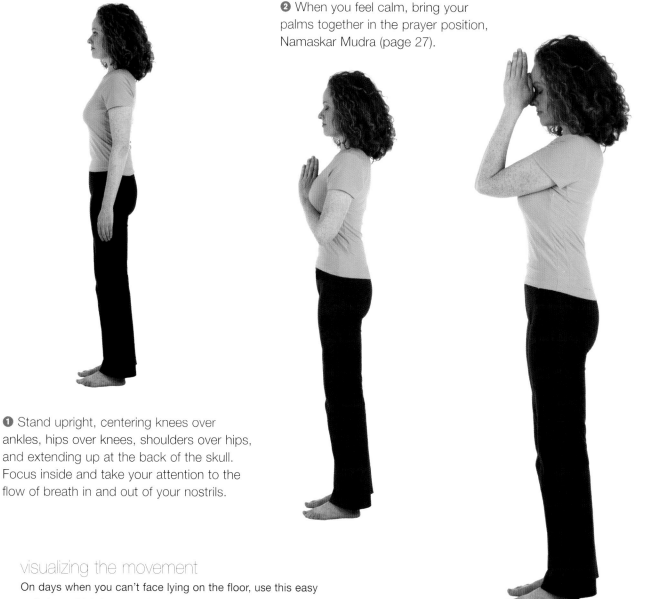

❷ When you feel calm, bring your palms together in the prayer position, Namaskar Mudra (page 27).

❶ Stand upright, centering knees over ankles, hips over knees, shoulders over hips, and extending up at the back of the skull. Focus inside and take your attention to the flow of breath in and out of your nostrils.

## visualizing the movement

On days when you can't face lying on the floor, use this easy variation, which features visualization and hand movements only. Make Namaskar Mudra as above, but open your palms slightly to leave a space that signifies offering. Then visualize yourself making the prostrations.

❸ Focus your mind, close your eyes, and touch the crown of your head, third eye area, throat, and the center of your chest with your joined thumbs.

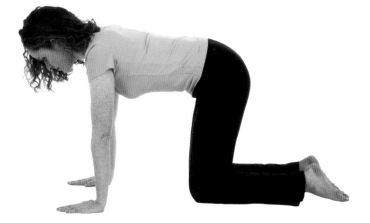

## holy lowliness

In Islam, the prostrations of prayer, especially bringing the face—the site of so many of the senses—and the essence of selfhood, the brain, to the floor, are a physical manifestation of submission that have a purifying effect, making men and women worthy of entering the realm of the divine. The prostration of mankind is likened in the Koran to the rising and setting of the sun, moon, and stars, all expressing humility in the face of God.

❹ Bend forward as if bowing. Bend your knees and come to a kneeling position, placing your palms on the floor.

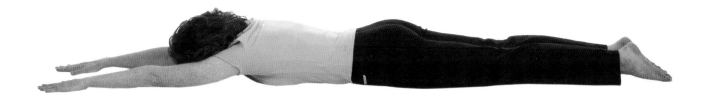

❺ Come forward, supported by your arms, and place your chest on the ground. Extend your arms in front of your head and rest your forehead on the floor. Stretch the legs away from the pelvis, heels and toes touching. Exhale your chest and shoulders down to the ground and let the floor support your hips and legs as if they were very heavy. Become absorbed in being as low as possible.

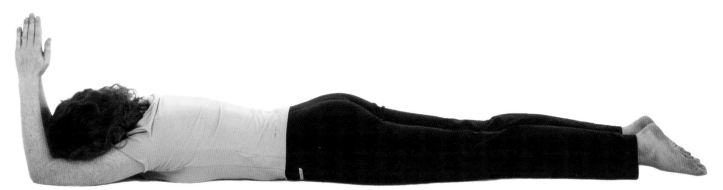

❻ Join your palms in prayer position again and bend your elbows to point your fingers at the sky. Get up and repeat the steps up to three times.

# whirling meditation

Some schools of yoga start sessions with some energy-clearing whirling. As you revolve on the spot, you spin off the concerns that preoccupied you before you entered the room, disorienting the senses in such a way that you start again with a clean slate. Dervishes from the Sufi path in Islam have a long tradition of whirling as a way of liberating body and mind from the material world and entering into a place in which there is no reality but the divine. You will need a wide, clear space in which to practice this transformative and life-affirming exercise. Don't worry if you start giggling.

❶ Stand with feet hip-width apart and focus on aligning your body. Establish a firm, stable base on all four parts of each foot (the base of the big and little toes and the sides of the heels). Then extend up through the ankles and legs, keeping the knees slightly bent. Pull the buttocks toward each other and tuck the abdomen back to support the lower spine. Lift out of the pelvis on both sides and stretch through both sides of the body equally. Broaden the chest as if opening a book and relax the shoulders away from the ears. Lengthen up the back of the neck, chin parallel to the floor and slightly tucked in.

❷ Focus on your breath, inhaling extension into the spine and exhaling stability into the feet. Take your gaze to one spot in front of you at eye level.

❸ Raise your arms at the side of your body to shoulder height, stretching away through the thumbs and little fingers. Start to turn to the left (the side of the body associated with the heart for Sufis and in yoga). Aim for seven spins at first, building up to twenty-one. Move the body first, the head last, and fix your gaze directly in front of you. Spin faster and faster until everything is a blur. If you feel too dizzy, stop.

❹ Settle yourself in the center again, then reverse the spinning action to the right. If you can't yet do twenty-one turns, don't worry; just go at your own pace and take the exercise as far as feels comfortable for you. After spinning, gently lower yourself to the ground and lie still, stretched out on your back as the world turns around you, and marvel at how invigorated yet quieted you feel.

## dizzy dancing

If you don't like the idea of spinning, yet want to stir yourself up, put on some music you love and just dance. Don't worry about set steps and great moves—no one's watching and there are no rules; just let the spirit move you.

"When I feel down, I put on some dance music and just go for it."

**Ken, driver**

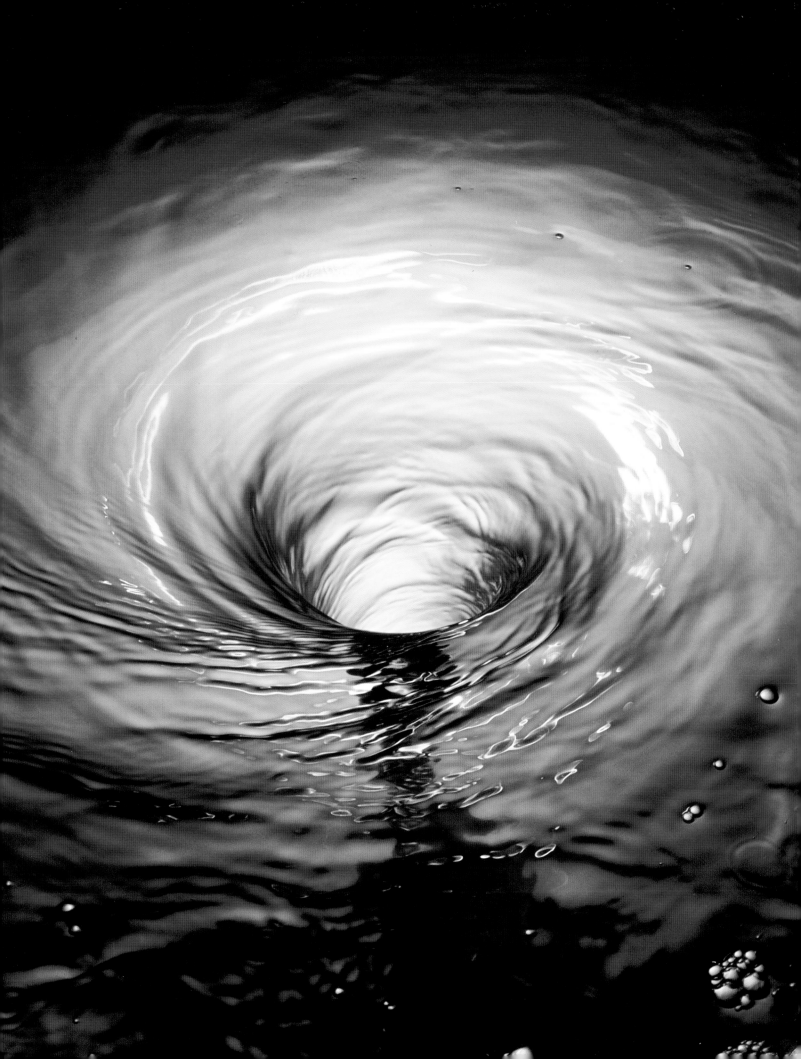

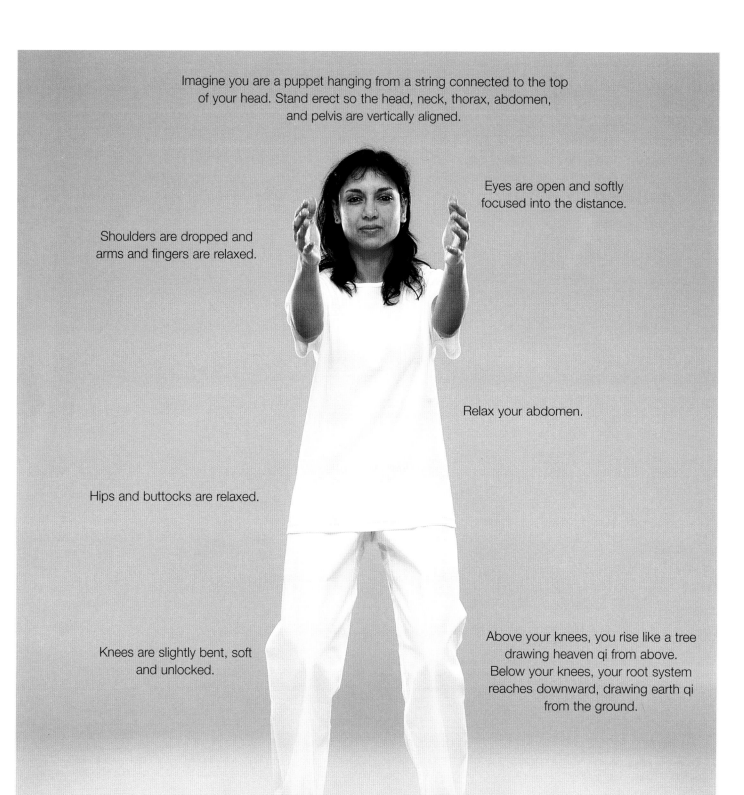

Imagine you are a puppet hanging from a string connected to the top
of your head. Stand erect so the head, neck, thorax, abdomen,
and pelvis are vertically aligned.

Eyes are open and softly
focused into the distance.

Shoulders are dropped and
arms and fingers are relaxed.

Relax your abdomen.

Hips and buttocks are relaxed.

Knees are slightly bent, soft
and unlocked.

Above your knees, you rise like a tree
drawing heaven qi from above.
Below your knees, your root system
reaches downward, drawing earth qi
from the ground.

Feet are hip-width apart.

# qi gong sequence

Like yoga, qi gong, the ancient Chinese form of energy exercise, uses movements of the body and breath practiced with mindfulness to balance subtle energies, promote the free-flow of the life force, qi, through vital energy channels, or meridians, and bring you into connection with the energy of the world around you. This not only promotes the well-being and self-repair of the body, it stills and opens the mind. Inhabiting the state of qi gong is to be relaxed and tranquil in body and mind. This standing exercise is meditation in motion; practitioners teach that as you work, you look but see nothing and listen but hear nothing until you no longer practice the movements, you embody them.

❶ Adopt the basic relaxed pose of qi gong: with feet a little more than hip-width apart and knees relaxed, let the shoulders drop forward and down, relax the armpits and elbows, drop back in the waist, and let the head and face be soft and loose. Hold for two minutes, keeping the mind free and relaxed.

❷ With knees still bent but extending out slightly, tilt the sacrum forward and extend the spine from the base up the back of the neck to the crown of the head.

❸ Raise your arms to shoulder height in front of you. Imagining you are balancing an orange beneath each armpit and a huge balloon in front of your chest, spread your fingertips slightly apart. Keep them level with the neck, palms facing in and curving inward, and make space between each digit. The arms form a relaxed oval.

❹ Keeping the back of the neck long, chin tucked in slightly, take your gaze into the distance. Hold, relaxing your shoulders and abdomen and emptying your mind for up to fifteen minutes. Try not to overengage your muscles; work instead with mental intention, the body existing in a state of relaxed tension. Feel warmth spreading out from your lower abdomen and energy flowing up into you from the ground. Don't worry if you start to sway gently.

## being upright

It is a central principle of qi gong to stand tall, for when physically upright we stay mentally engaged and contented. As in Zen meditation, when the body adopts a posture, you automatically take on the correct state of mind.

"I get all sorts of buzzing and tingling in my spine and fingers when I practice energy exercises. Then I know I'm getting back in touch with myself."

Jane, critic

# walking with mindfulness

When walking with focus, it becomes possible even in the most mundane of situations—while window-shopping, between meetings—to refocus thoughts and energies by doing nothing but following the pace with the mind as it coordinates with the flow of breaths in and out. Walking with awareness is a tried-and-true meditative technique that has formed part of spiritual pilgrimages across the world since earliest times. Let the energies of the natural world retune you as you walk: if you feel flighty, focus on the stable earth beneath your feet; when your brain feels fuzzy, bring your attention to your head in the clouds. You might like to combine this exercise with the nature meditation on pages 74–75.

❶ As you start walking, your gait steady, spine straight, and gaze fixed up and slightly ahead, drift away from your thoughts and all notions of arriving and destination. Instead, tune in to your breathing.

❷ After a while, notice how your in and out breaths naturally fall in time with your pace. Watch how your whole body is brought into the walking action: your shoulders, hands, and hips, as well as your feet and legs.

❸ Start to slow your pace and begin to experience walking in awareness. Become conscious of every movement. Without looking at your feet, see them lifting and being replaced on the ground. Be aware of your knees flexing and straightening. Notice which part of the foot touches the floor first. Feel the weight transfer forward from your heel to the ball of your foot and then to the toes. Sense the suppleness of your body and your innate sense of balance as your weight switches from side to side.

❹ Now switch your focus to your breathing, inhaling for two paces and exhaling for two paces. When thoughts of where you're going or where you came from intrude, come back to pure awareness of your pace and your breath. Feel your mind as steady as your constant pace until you are doing nothing but walking with awareness. Aim to walk for twenty minutes or more.

## destination meditation

Short walks are good for a quick mind-refreshment break, and a lunch break in the city can be as beneficial as an afternoon in the countryside. Map out a circular route if the terrain is poor for walking: you might use churches or mosques as spiritual reminders to focus within, or restaurants to jog your memory back to the mind food of meditation.

Hikes are probably best for meditation. When physical endurance occupies the body to the exclusion of thoughts and when you are within the glories of nature—fields, hills, wide beaches—it becomes hard to see where you end and the world begins.

Or try a swimming meditation; be mindful of each stroke, letting it bring your mind into the present, and allow the repetitive nature of the action to draw you away from distractions. Set yourself a time limit or a set number of laps to swim. A plus is that your body gets toned too.

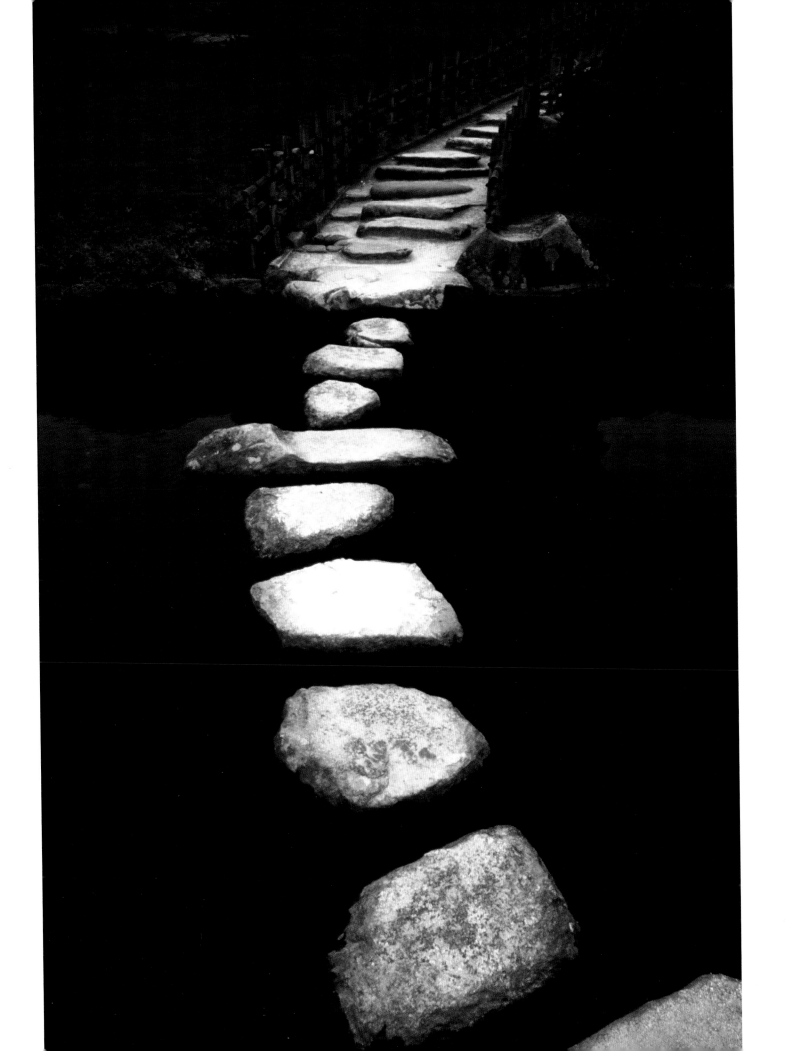

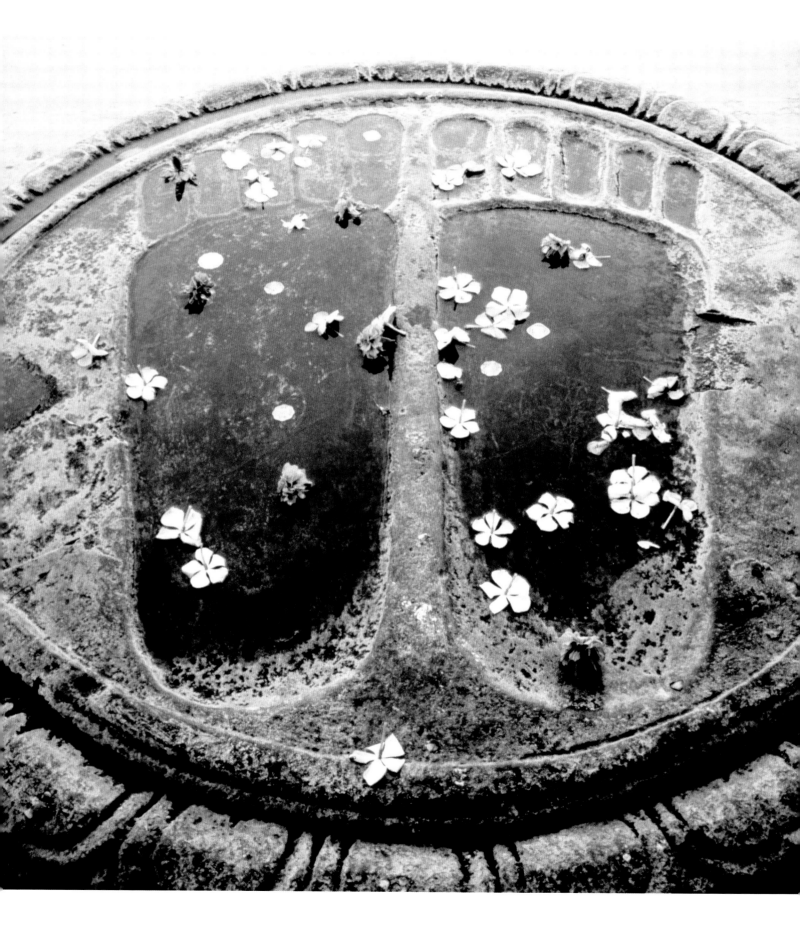

# just walking

*Kinhin* is zazen (pages 40–41) in motion. In Zen monasteries, monks walk very slowly, maintaining the meditation posture adopted during zazen with the upper body and processing in a clockwise direction around the altar in the meditation hall. Vipassana monasteries in Southeast Asia are built with a terrace for walking meditation. The changing movements of the body serve as a way of recalling the essentially transitory nature of life as well as exemplifying the notion that when one can find calmness in activity one is truly calm. This is a good way to get your mind in order for seated meditation, and is also effective when you want to continue meditating, but your legs and feet have fallen asleep while sitting or kneeling. You will need enough space to be able to take about thirty paces in a straight line. Walk barefooted if possible.

❶ Standing still at the start of your walking track, consciously lengthen your spine from the base to the top of your head. Imagine you are suspended by a string from the crown of your head. Make a soft fist with your left hand and place it in the center of your chest in line with your heart. Cover your left fist with your right hand, thumb resting over the top. Keep your elbows out, forearms parallel to the floor. Alternatively, adopt one of the mudras on pages 26–27. Center yourself by closing your eyes and witnessing your breath moving in and out.

❷ Open your eyes and look down and slightly forward, softening your gaze. Shift your left foot forward with an inhalation. Exhale. On the next inhalation step your right foot forward.

❸ Continue along your path at this slow pace. Just walk; do nothing else—watch your breathing or count the paces if you need to focus your mind. When thoughts intrude, let them rise, acknowledge them, and let them go. Do not admonish yourself; simply return to the act of walking.

❹ Work calmly and steadily for ten to twenty minutes, your upper body held as if seated for meditation, and only your lower body moving. Be aware simply of the repetitious action of each foot lifting, moving forward, lowering to the ground, and transferring weight from heel to toe.

## a private pilgrimage

Like an extended walking meditation, a spiritual pilgrimage is traditionally undertaken on foot. The Christian journey to Santiago de Compostela in Spain, the Muslim Hajj in Mecca, and the Buddhist's journey to the birthplace of Siddhartha Gautama at Bodhgaya share the notion that as you draw nearer to the holy site with each step, you progress further along the journey away from ignorance and shortsightedness. The real journey makes physical the intangible as the body makes flesh the will of the spirit. The physical privations of the long journey only serve to magnify the pilgrim's spiritual development. You might plan a walk to a spiritual site that has resonance for you. Whether it is the parish church in the next town or a prominent hill out in the countryside, the journeying is as valuable a part of the experience as the arrival; some would argue it is more important. Think of it as a double path, leading you inside as well as to the place of worship.

**left:** Sacred sites across Asia known as "Buddha's footprints" (this one is in India) have become places of pilgrimage.

# gardening with mindfulness

Gardening is therapeutic. When faced with heartbreak, illness, or uncertainty, many people retreat outside to lose themselves in mechanical digging, weeding, and pruning. As you concentrate only on the physical task at hand, you find peace, stillness, and a broadness of perception. Nurturing plants and watching them flourish and fight disease can become a purposeful passion charged with optimism. Walk around a garden 365 days a year and each time you'll spot something new, something that wasn't there hours before. Gardening keeps you in the present and aware of the movement of time, of the state of flux that is the seasons and the revolving planet. Whether your garden is a scented window box overlooking a busy road or an oasis of calm in the country, you can use this meditation.

❶ As you perform your tasks in the garden, lose yourself in the work. When weeding, focus only on the bed, the plants, and the action of pulling or chasing roots. When digging, savor the repetitive actions of hands and feet and the turning of the soil. When pruning, take your gaze to each stem in turn, deciding where to make the cut.

❷ As thoughts propel your mind along other avenues, watch yourself being pulled this way and that by judgment, desire, and emotions. Let them be, and return to the task at hand. Stay quiet inside.

❸ Notice the signatures of the seasons and learn to appreciate the ever-changing, glorious impermanence of a garden, where every spring marks a new start and renewed possibilities of perfection.

❹ Consider the cyclical nature of life in seeds, flowers, pods, and compost. Tune in to the complexity of connections between health and disease, predators and bugs, life and death. Ponder your role as nurturer and destroyer. Think about the life of the garden after your time.

❺ Make yours a twenty-four-hour garden. At night, enjoy moonlight on silver leaves; in the evening, stop to appreciate night-scented blooms. Let your garden attract all the senses with swishing grasses and tinkling fountains, hidden arbors, and scents for every time of day.

❻ In the end, find yourself performing daily tasks not just for the material rewards of fruit and flowers, shade and scent, but because the act of gardening brings you into a state of inner contentment and outer connection with the world.

## "When my father died, nurturing the garden for the first time eased my anger and gave me hope."

Khadija, lawyer

### getting to know your garden

Use this sense meditation to get in touch with the life in your garden. You will need a tree or two. Ask a friend to blindfold you in the garden and lead you to a tree. Use your senses to get to know the tree. Feel the texture of the bark with your fingers and cheek. Put your ear to the trunk and be astonished by the ticking and whooshing within; really smell the wood. Ask your friend to lead you away from the tree. Take off the blindfold and try to identify the tree.

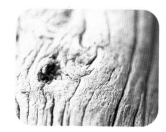

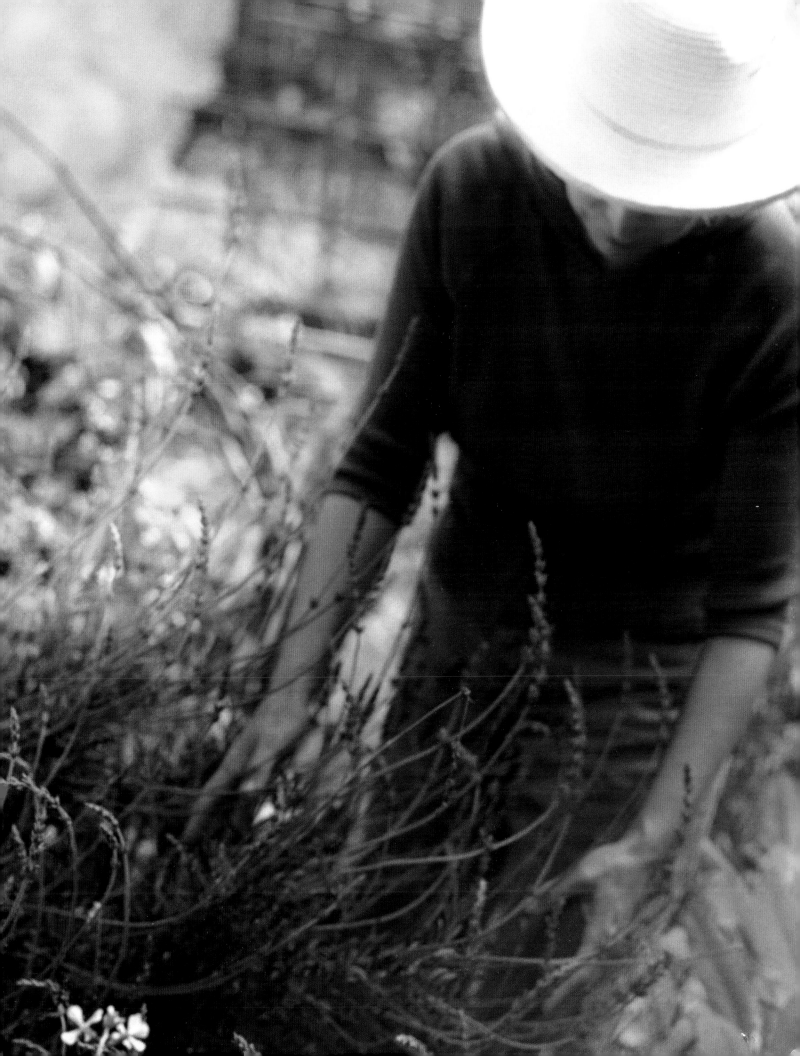

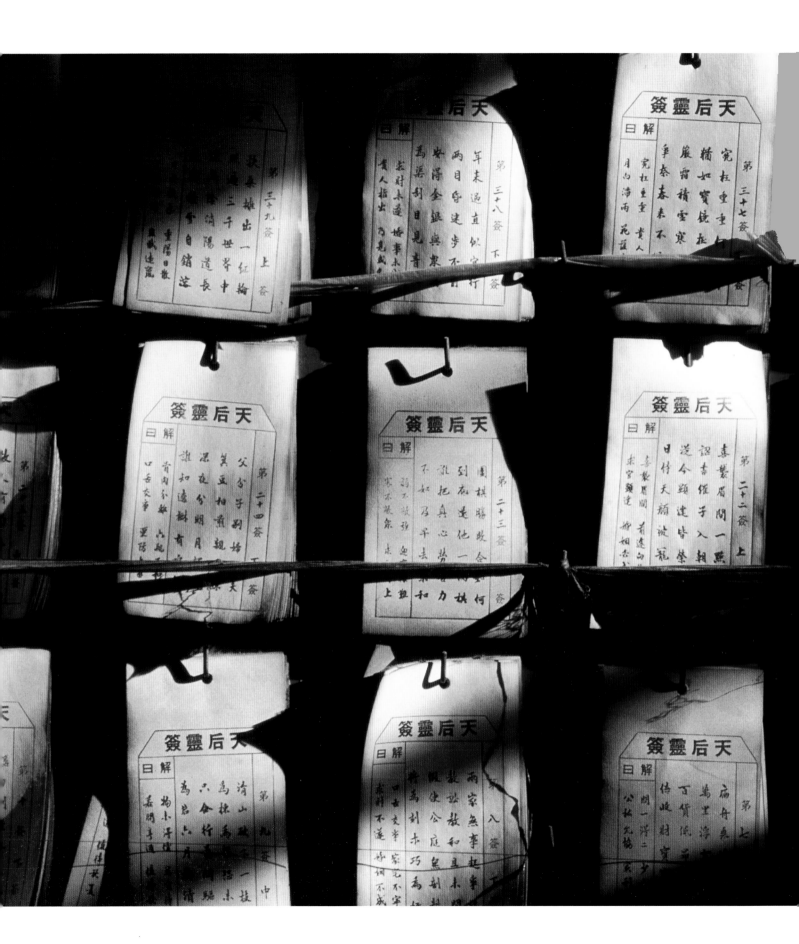

# the art of calligraphy

Calligraphy developed as an art form in China thousands of years ago and the results are mindfulness visualized. Each mark becomes a permanent expression of the calligrapher's nature, as well as the essence of a word. Contemplate single-word examples of calligraphy as a meditation, trying to glean the essence of the strokes. Often the movement and intensity of the strokes make the meanings of words such as "speed," "grace," or "strength" startlingly self-evident. Alternatively, use this writing exercise to bring mindfulness to your own hand. You will need a pen and paper.

❶ Sit comfortably upright (pages 22–24), extending the spine upward from the tailbone to the crown of the head. Take the pen and hold it in the same way. Japanese calligraphy students are taught that to have a slanting pen or back will be reflected in the mind, which remains unfocused.

❷ Relax with each out breath, keep the pen balanced in a state of relaxed tension, and quiet the mind. Start to write—you might work with your name or the words "peace," "happiness," or "mindfulness."

❸ Write the word over and over, letting the repetition absolve you from the need to be creative or think. Let your personality shine through each stroke and try to pick up what this says about your nature. Stand back from yourself to witness the distance between your action and yourself.

## writing mantras

The meditation known as *likhita japa* in Sanskrit involves repeatedly writing mantras. The unique energy charge of the word is invoked and released as you repeatedly write it in tiny script. Work over and over with the spoken examples on pages 120–21, releasing the essence of the letters and imbuing yourself with the spiritual energy of each word.

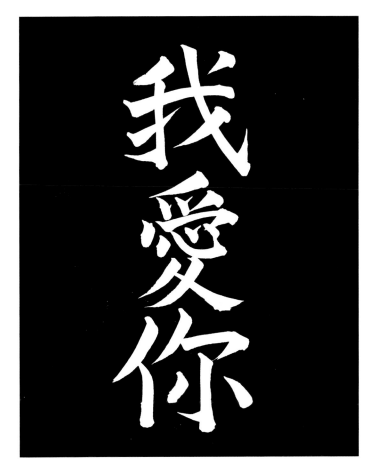

## illuminating the heart

Early Celtic Christian texts such as the *Book of Kells* show draftsmanship made a fine art. Scribes spent up to a year painstakingly transcribing the words of the Bible and other holy writings, speaking the words aloud as they wrote in an act of mindfulness that can be likened to mantra recitation. The words are decorated with abstract, geometric motifs. Labyrinthine ribbons lace in and out and never-ending spirals lead the eye into the interior, their intricate twists and turns representing the infinite options and brain-twisting confusion of choices for those on the spiritual path. Rose motifs symbolize the rose garden, a quiet place within to retreat for contemplation and inner transformation. Such illuminations created in an act of meditation shed light on the spirit of the worker while offering the viewer a pathway to peace.

# shower power

Cleansing the spirit comes easily in the shower, where purifying water rains down and the body is at its most elemental, without the distraction of clothing and makeup. Before their morning ablutions, Zen monks pledge, "I must cleanse my body and my heart." Make cleansing the body an essential part of your own daily devotion each morning or evening by expressing the intention to become pure as you use this transformative, exfoliative meditation. You will need a couple handfuls of sea salt moistened to a paste with warm water.

❶ As you shed your clothes and wipe away makeup, divest yourself of your pretensions and preconceptions, too. State your intention to stand before yourself free from artifice.

❷ Stepping into the shower, celebrate the cleansing potential of the earth's life-giving element, water. Let the power of the jet wash away concerns. Pledge to become like water, ever-changing but always true to its nature.

❸ Take handfuls of the salt scrub and massage it into the skin, starting at your heels and moving up the body, making large circles in the direction of the heart. As you slough off the dead skin cells, sense the infinite options of new beginnings. Rinse off with the shower.

❹ Start to wash with soap—try sandalwood for spiritual inspiration and a heavenly scent. As you cleanse each part of your body, bring your attention to its function. Give thanks and promise to use it only for good deeds.

❺ Finish with a blast of invigoratingly cold water to bring your senses back into the now. After patting the skin dry, anoint your body with a refreshing and uplifting body oil. Mix four or five drops in total of rose, patchouli, or sandalwood oil into two teaspoons of sweet almond oil, shake well, then massage into the skin.

## spring into life

Hot springs have been adopted as a source of spiritual sustenance as well as of relaxation and cleansing across many cultures. In Japan, daily bathing in the natural springs—*onsen*—that dot the countryside offers a chance for peace, solitude, and reflection alongside the ritual cleansing that is key to the Shinto religion. Often fed by mountain streams, onsen are sited in breathtaking natural settings, which serve to inspire and enlighten the spirit during meditation. Waterfalls are considered especially auspicious in these purification and meditation rites. To gain the same effect, sit upright and listen to a waterfall or fountain (a CD will suffice if you really can't get outside). Take your focus to the sound, letting it fill your ears. Close your eyes if it helps. Listen for patterns in the constant flow, for brief silences amid the bubbles and crackles. Take the sounds inside, allowing them to fuse with the flow of blood and fluids within your body.

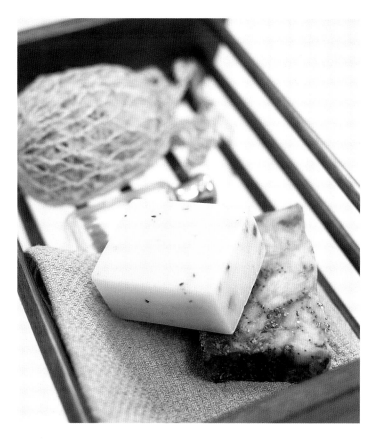

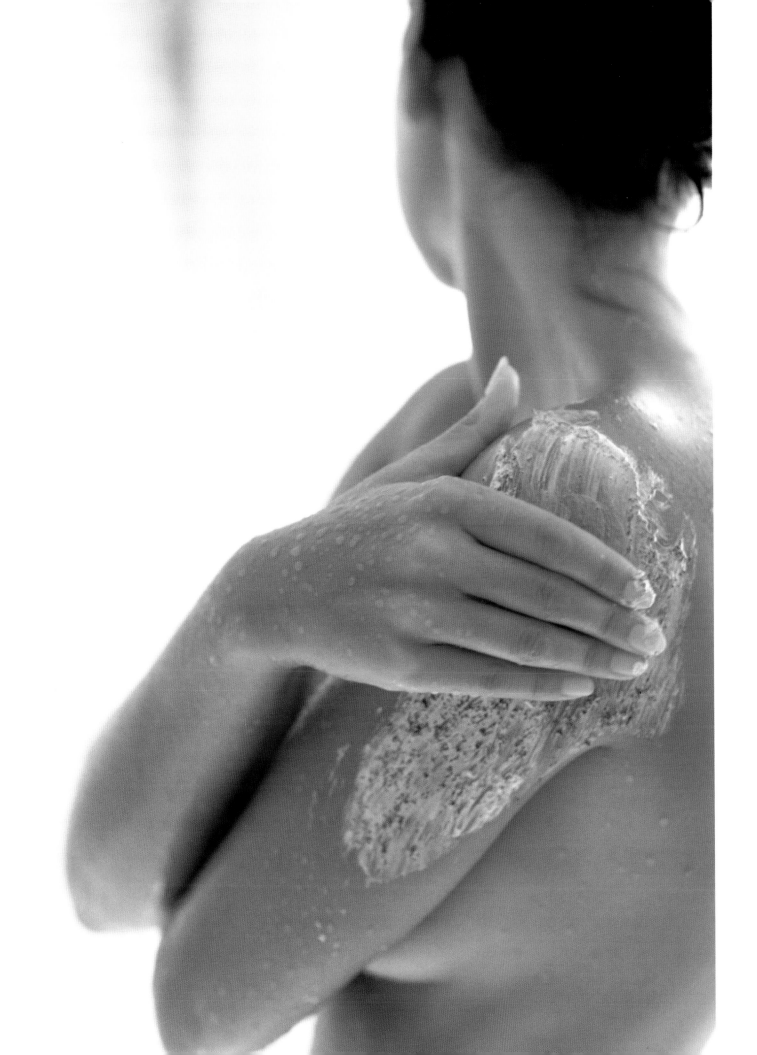

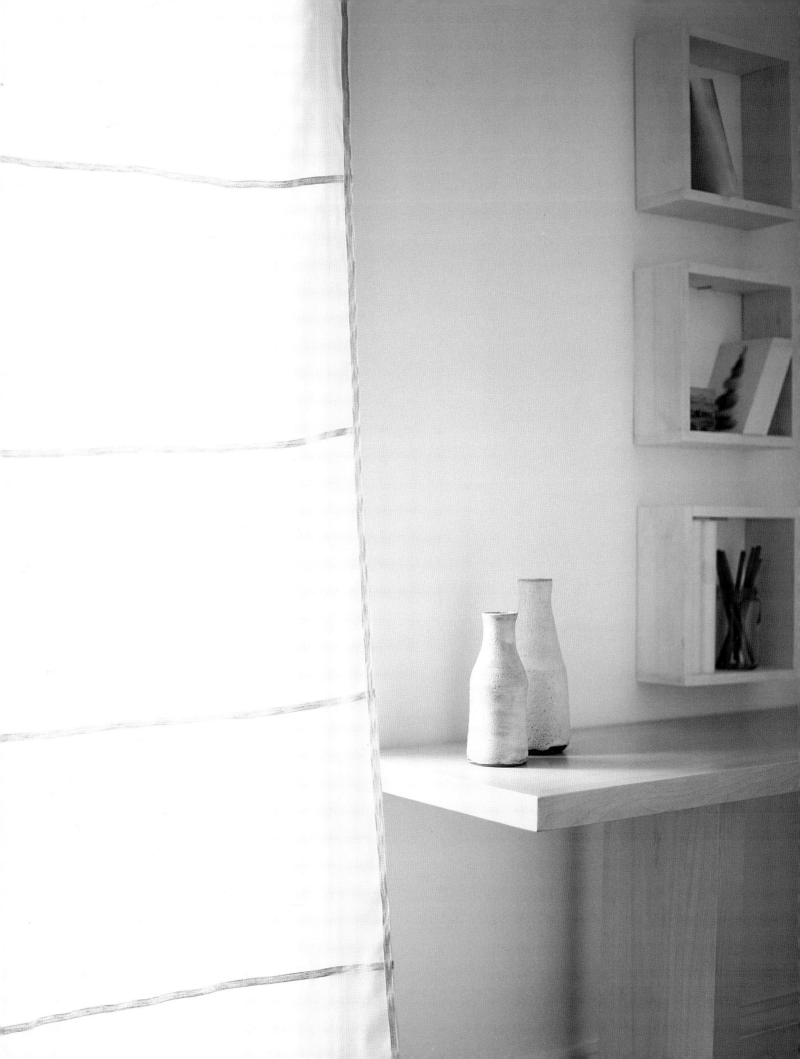

# clutter clearing

Clutter fills your space with emotions and expectations that distract you from the present. That box of old love letters, piles of clothes that no longer fit, broken china, and files of work that you really should be doing are physical manifestations of regret, delusion, and obligation that tie you to the past and indebt you to the future. Who wants to cohabit with those kinds of ghosts? Use this clutter-clearing meditation to bring you back in line with what's important right here, right now. Let this mindful activity simplify your life so you can respond fully to the present and fill your space with only those items that promise mental and physical freedom.

❶ Sit comfortably and decide what you want to get out of the exercise. Write it down. Aside from the obvious—more space and less dust—it might be to set the seal on a past relationship or to find a new direction in your career.

❷ Target one room at a time for clutter clearing, setting aside more time than you think you need and blocking it out in your schedule. Don't be distracted. When the time comes, settle into the activity, switching off your mind by focusing on the physical actions of clearing, sorting, dusting, and throwing away.

❸ Start at one corner of the room and move methodically through the space. With every object you meet, disengage your mind from emotional responses, from the memories it stirs up, and from the obligations it represents. Simply ask yourself, "How will this help me get what I want (a new relationship, better career, cleaner room)?" If you're aiming for a promotion, for example, you might jettison all the work clothes that don't make you feel authoritative, capable, and enterprising.

❹ Set aside a bag for the thrift store, a bag for trash, a bag for items that you can burn ceremonially to honor the past and mark the transformation of difficult feelings into clearer ways of seeing. You should be left with just a small bag for items that have earned their place in your new space.

❺ As you work, repeat a mantra to remind you of your purpose. It might be "Leave no stone unturned" or "Pure space." When you come across difficult boxes and piles, those that force you to confront distressing issues, such as divorce, death, and guilt, keep returning to witness mode, trying to note from a distance the effect these objects and the emotions tied to them have on you. Learn more about your relation to the world and those things that may be standing in the way of your progression.

❻ As you clear the space, sweep, dust, and wipe clean with refreshingly fragranced cleaning fluids. Feel your own slate being wiped clean as you leave behind the past and start to inhabit the present.

❼ Rearrange your space using only those items that make your life feel lighter, clearer, and more purposeful. Give prominence to objects of beauty that connote happiness and peace.

## living with awareness

When you can make meditation part of everyday life, you find real peace. Being able to switch off from the madness of work and family life and focus on something mechanical saves lives. In this state of passive activity you reconnect with the heart and switch off the mind as you retreat from the world and connect with the ebb and flow of reality.

# cleaning meditation

If you hate housework, cleaning your home can offer a fine opportunity for mindfulness. Use the time you usually begrudge to work with attention as you dust and vacuum, polish and mop. As you work, you clear away sloth and lethargy, some of the most common hindrances to meditation practice. The result? A cleansed mind fit for your scrubbed, clutter-free home.

❶ Once a week, set aside an hour to clean your home. Turn off the radio and television and take the phone off the hook. Then gather together everything you need: bucket and mop, water and detergent, vacuum cleaner, duster and polish. Before you start cleaning, center yourself by standing upright and watching your breath move in and out. Close your eyes if it helps.

❷ As you sweep and polish, scrub and clear away, engage fully with the actions. Don't rush them or scrimp; keep your mind on the matter at hand. Fully experience every sweep of the hand and flick of the wrist. Eventually you will notice your breath linking in with the actions.

❸ Whenever you find thoughts and feelings grabbing the limelight, take a step back and become conscious of them. Think about their underlying emotional tone; don't look at the particular thoughts, but at what underpins them—perhaps worry, unhappiness, excitement—consider briefly how these emotions might hinder your progress in meditation. Don't get stuck in them, but keep coming back to the very physical act you are engaged in.

❹ When the time is up, put away your cleaning supplies. Look around your home and see how much more welcoming and easy to live in it feels. Sense an equivalent clearheadedness and feel how full of energy you are, how alert your body is.

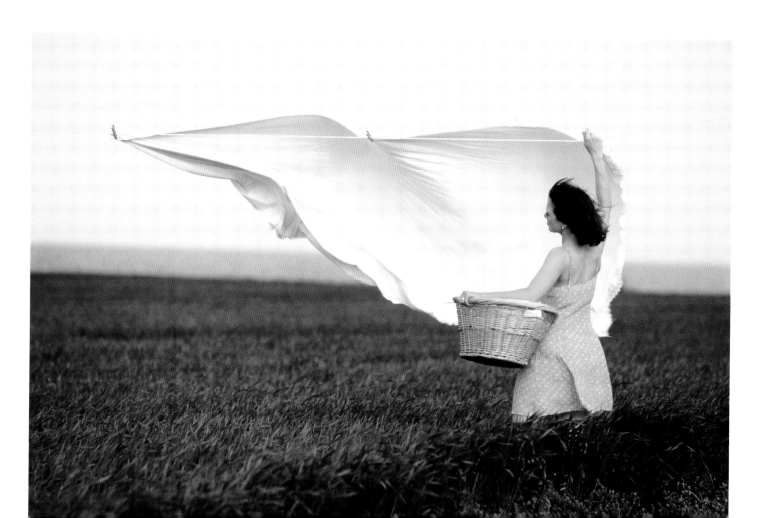

## conserving energy

When you feel assaulted by sensations and emotions as a result of clearing the clutter and cleaning your home, retreat to a safe place for a while by performing the yoga posture Kadapidasana, or the Ear-closing Pose, which shuts down the senses. If you find this advanced pose too much of a challenge, kneel on your heels and then place your thumbs in your ears, fingers over your eyes, and bend forward to rest your chest on your thighs, forehead on the floor.

**1** Lie on your back, arms by your sides, palms down, knees bent. Bring your knees toward your chest and push down with your arms to lift your legs into the air. Straightening your legs, take them beyond your head and rest your feet on their tiptoes, heels stretching away. Feel an intense stretch in the upper back and let your chest compress your chin into your throat. Stretch your arms along the floor behind you and hold the posture (Halasana, or the Plow Pose) for a while, inhaling deep in the abdomen.

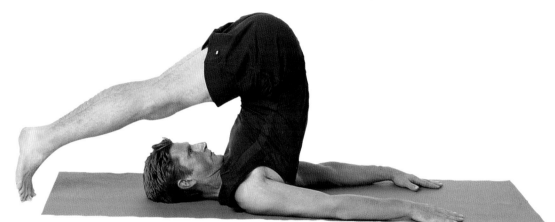

**2** Bend your knees and draw them toward your shoulders, blocking your ears. Close your eyes and focus on your breath.

**3** Fold your arms around the back of your knees, clasping the opposite forearms. Let your mind drift for thirty seconds or more. Release the arms and curl down, vertebra by vertebra, on an exhalation.

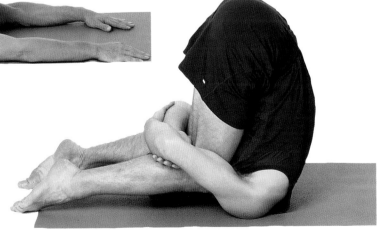

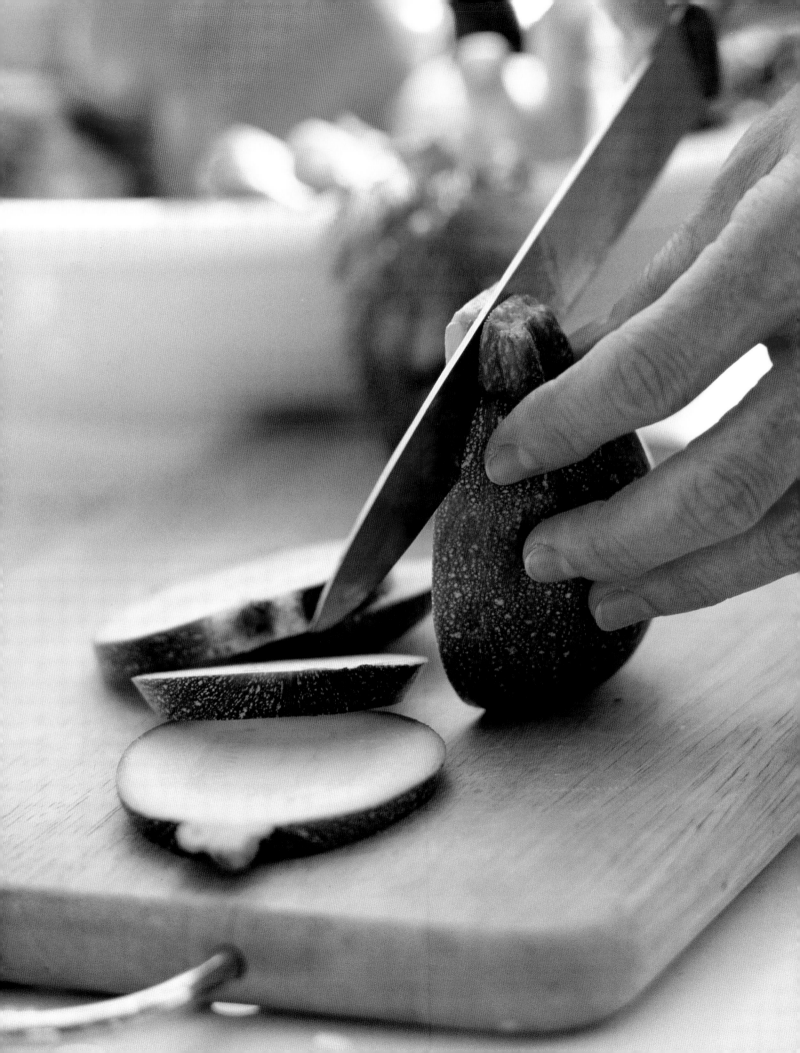

# conscious cooking

Most people can't be bothered to cook meals from scratch each day: fast food accounts for the largest slice of consumer spending on food. Yet dishes prepared with love and thoughtful attention from carefully selected fresh ingredients nourish the spirit of those who concoct them as well as the health of those who dine on them. Cooking is an experience of transformation that we should—like Zen monks—consider a great honor to take part in. Magic happens when foods from different life sources are turned by chopping and heat into something capable of sustaining human life. Bring some of this magic into your kitchen with this meditation.

❶ Leave your preoccupations and worries at the kitchen door. As you wash your hands, imagine the day's concerns being rinsed away with the physical dirt and impurities. Wipe over work surfaces in the same frame of mind.

❷ Bring together all your ingredients. Handle them carefully as the offerings of other life sources. State your intention to increase the happiness of those you are cooking for. Declare it out loud, if you like.

❸ Let the activities of washing, chopping, and stirring suffuse your body and mind. Surrender yourself to each task, letting it be an outward sign of your inward state—calm, untroubled by distractions, and full of love.

❹ As your mind gets drawn away by thoughts, constantly anchor yourself to the task at hand and to your intention—to satisfy with good food and love.

❺ As you work, visualize the food you are preparing nourishing the diners with love, and see this love spreading out from the dining table as they take it with them out into their own lives and interactions.

❻ Present the food beautifully—not with carved vegetables and florid napkins, but by honestly and mindfully placing it on the plate. Now, even before it is eaten, the recipient will absorb feelings of caring and emotional sustenance.

## kitchen karma

*Vaastu*, the Indian art of placement, suggests that food is best prepared facing east, the direction associated with the sun. On the Vaastu Purusha mandala, the blueprint used to impose harmony and order on an interior design, the Vedic sun god Surya rules over the eastern quadrant of a space, representing physical light and spiritual enlightenment. To prepare food in this part of a home, therefore, brings you into confluence with these qualities and imbues your food with inspiration.

"First thing in the morning I'm at my happiest, cooking breakfast with loud music and everything just flowing—nice butter, good ingredients, hungry children."

**Jonny, caregiver**

# baking bread

Alive with yeast, bread is enveloped in ideas of spiritual sustenance. Across the globe, this staff of life is marked with the sign of the cross, included on the Sabbath table, and revered as a divine gift. The act of kneading the living dough when attended to with care and mindfulness draws you into communion with this spiritual charge. Use this recipe when you want to get connected with yourself and partake in some of the spiritual succor of this elemental food.

❶ Assemble all the ingredients (see box). Tie on an apron, taking on as you do a sense of occasion. Wash your hands, imagining your preoccupations being rinsed away with the dirt of the day. Vow to work mindfully, paying attention to nothing but the breadmaking process.

❷ Pour the yeast into a small bowl and add about a fourth of the water. Leave to dissolve for 5 minutes. In a large mixing bowl, combine the flour and salt. Make a well in the center and add the foaming yeast mixture.

❸ Use a wooden spoon to draw in flour from the side of the bowl little by little to make a stiff paste. Then add the rest of the water a little at a time, bringing in the flour until you have a sticky but firm mass. Let the stirring erase all thoughts from your mind.

❹ Tip the doughy mass onto a floured surface. Start to knead, using the heel of your hand, adding more flour as necessary. As you work, the starches in the flour will begin to break down to feed the yeast. Ponder this transformation and nourishment.

❺ Knead with your whole body, not just your hands. Stand up, take a few deep breaths, lengthening the exhalation, then start the movement at your shoulders. As you work, let it broaden your chest, allowing the lungs to expand fully. Feel any knots and tight muscles in the shoulders and neck easing as the dough becomes more springy and silklike. Work for 10 minutes.

❻ Place the dough in a clean, oiled bowl and cover with a clean dishcloth. Leave to stand at room temperature until doubled in size, 1 1/2–2 hours.

## basic bread recipe

Ingredients:

2 tsp. dried yeast • 11 fl. oz. lukewarm water
• 1 lb. strong white bread flour • 2 tsp. salt

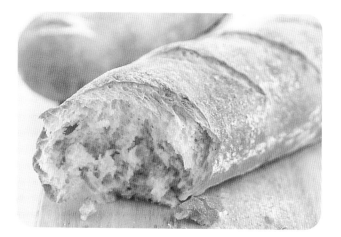

❼ Knock back the dough by punching it with your knuckles. Let it rest for 10 minutes. Turn onto a floured board and form into an even round, rotating it as you work. Place on a floured cookie sheet and leave to proof (double in size) in a warm place for 35–45 minutes. Preheat the oven to 425°F.

❽ Slash the top of the loaf with a sharp knife and bake for 45–50 minutes, until golden brown and hollow when tapped on the bottom. Leave to cool on a wire rack before cutting. Serve with pride and love.

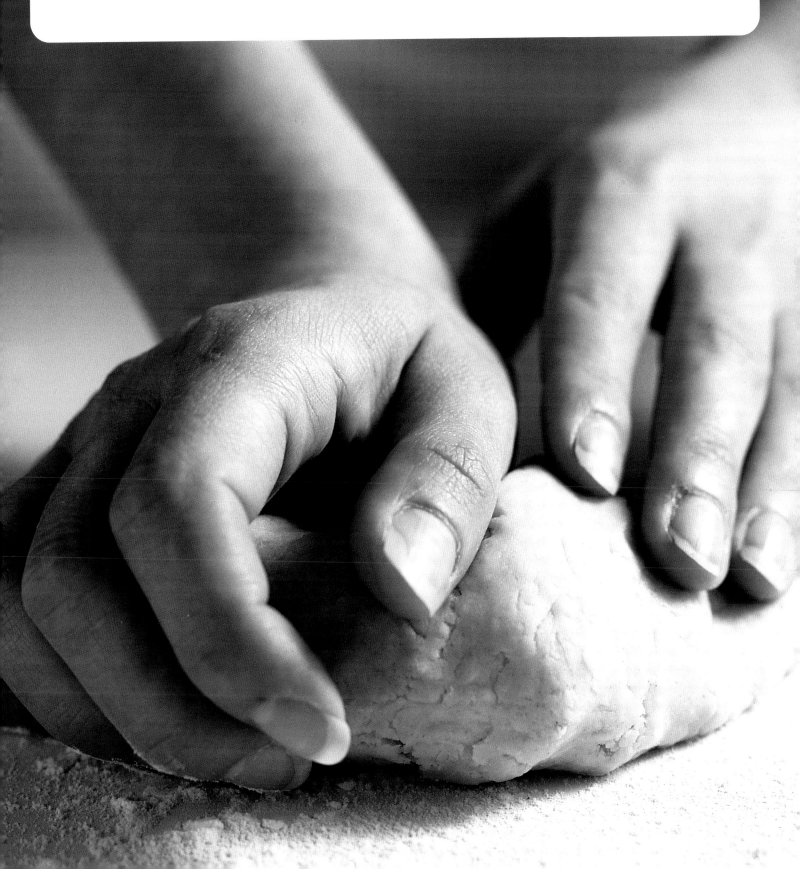

"I don't bake every day, just for special occasions, but when I do it's deeply satisfying."

Tina, accountant

"Because it is empty, the sage's mind can receive.
Because it is still, it can respond."
**Hui Tsang**

# breath meditation

- **Counting the breath**
- **Lengthening the breath**
- **So-ham meditation**
- **Alternate-nostril breathing**

When you pay attention to your breath, you are meditating. Inevitably, as you watch the inflow and exit of air though your nostrils, as you feel the diaphragm move up and down and the rib cage expand, you are witnessing the present moment and excluding everything else from your thoughts. This is inner peace, and it is this easy to find. Learning to listen to, harness, and refine the breath is considered in yoga so important to personal evolution that pranayama, or breath control, is one of the eight limbs, or steps, on the yoga ladder to moksha, freedom from the material world. In the Anapanasati Sutta, the Buddha teaches that breathing with full awareness is the first stage in "the perfect accomplishment of true understanding and complete liberation." The pages that follow introduce yoga techniques that use your awareness to control your breathing, quieting your mind and revitalizing your body while you suffuse yourself with prana, the energy of life.

# counting the breath

Paying attention during meditation is difficult. Having a focus for your thoughts keeps them from running away from the act of simply sitting. Try this breath-counting exercise to ease yourself into the breathing meditations. If you prefer a physical focus to keep your mind on the straight and narrow, start with the pebble-counting exercise on page 42.

❶ Sit or kneel comfortably upright, hands resting on knees or thighs (pages 22–27). Close your eyes. Settle yourself by watching your breath moving in and out for a moment. Feel your rib cage expand with the inhalation, and the coolness on your upper lip during the exhalation.

❷ When you feel calm and your breathing has steadied and deepened, start counting: silently say "One" on the first in breath and "One" on the first out breath. Continue counting in this way, seeing how far you can get without your attention wandering from the number. Never force the breath: keep everything really relaxed.

❸ Once your thoughts wander, return to awareness of your breath and start again. At first you may only get to two, but with perseverance and steady practice you will hit ten or more. Whatever number you reach, see how, by stilling the breath, you become absorbed inside, calm and alert.

❹ Keep coming back to this exercise as you become more practiced at meditation, seeing how far you can progress without thoughts, sensations, or emotions distracting your focus. Some teachers set a tough target of the auspicious number 108.

## assessing your progress

Every couple of months, take ten minutes or so to look at your progress in meditation. Sit down in a quiet place and focus your mind by watching your breathing, as if starting to meditate. When you feel quiet, reflect on your meditation. Are the techniques becoming easier? Is the meditation changing your daily life? Has your concentration span lengthened? Are your relationships at work less fraught? Are panic and stress being replaced, if not by calmness, then at least by an awareness of how you react to stressful situations? Congratulate yourself on how far you've come and start thinking about where you want to go.

## thought monitoring

Try to be aware of thoughts the moment they occur, not after some moments of daydreaming. As you work with meditation, your perception of intrusive thoughts will sharpen and become more penetrating. Keep your focus keen.

"Every night when the house is quiet, I come back to my sewing for half an hour or so. By counting as I stitch I keep my mind as sharp as the needle."

Karen, interior designer

# lengthening the breath

The cleansing yoga breathing technique Khumbhaka teaches you how to lengthen your breathing pattern so that the out breath extends, offering you opportunity to cleanse yourself from the inside out. Use it before starting a sitting meditation when you feel particularly "impure"—you have a hangover or haven't been behaving as well as you should. This technique also includes a pause, interrupting the breath so you experience the power of stillness amid the flow.

❶ Sit comfortably upright, hands resting on knees or thighs (pages 22–27). Close your eyes and focus on the movement in and out of your regular breathing pattern. Notice the breath cool as you inhale and warm as you exhale.

❷ Inhale to a count of four. Pause, retaining the breath for a count of four, then exhale for four. This is one cycle. Take a regular breath if necessary. Repeat three, five, or seven cycles. Work with this technique for a few weeks.

❸ When you feel comfortable with the technique, start to lengthen the out breath. Inhale for four, pause for a count of four, and exhale to the count of eight. Take a regular breath, if necessary. On the exhalation, let calmness envelop you, then let the in breath come naturally and easily. As you pause, retaining the breath, do not tense or let the shoulders rise, but feel a sense of still, profound clarity and spaciousness. Work for three to five minutes, settling into a constant and easy rhythm.

## reading and doing

It's great to read about meditation, but you learn most from doing, simply sitting and turning within. If you're finding it hard to get down to the practicalities of meditation, set yourself some simple targets—perhaps sitting to meditate for five minutes twice a week. Then, release yourself from guilt trips. The more you practice, the more you'll want to practice.

## visualization

After some weeks, when the technique feels perfectly natural, start to add a purifying visualization technique to the exhalation. With the extended out breath, exhale all your negativity, impurities, stagnant energy, and unhelpful emotions; on the in breath, imagine happiness, peace, and vitality suffusing you from the toes up. Work for five minutes, then sit quietly, savoring the refreshing sense of rejuvenation.

"If you would swim on the bosom of the ocean of Truth, you must reduce yourself to a zero."

Mahatma Gandhi

# so-ham meditation

This incredibly easy and centuries-old breathing technique takes your focus simultaneously within and without while anchoring you in the present. With each in breath you repeat the word "So"; on the out breath you say "Ham." It's that simple, and you can speak out loud, whisper the words, or repeat them silently. What is so profound about this simple technique is the meaning of the words: "So" signifies oneself and is said to be the sound made by every living creature when inhaling; "Ham" refers to the universe and is the sound all creatures make when exhaling. And so in repeating the two words over and over with the inhalation and exhalation of prana, the life energy, you link yourself with the energy of the world and every living thing in it.

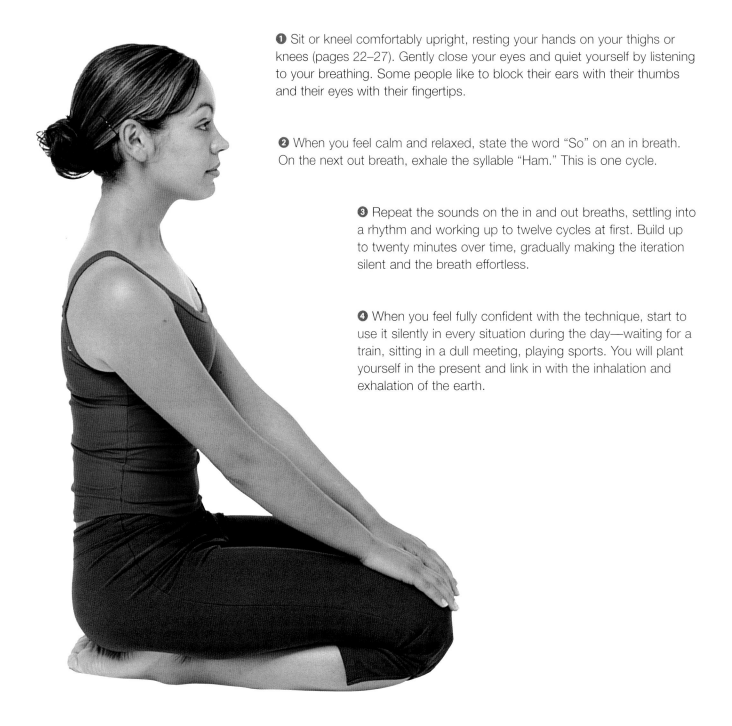

❶ Sit or kneel comfortably upright, resting your hands on your thighs or knees (pages 22–27). Gently close your eyes and quiet yourself by listening to your breathing. Some people like to block their ears with their thumbs and their eyes with their fingertips.

❷ When you feel calm and relaxed, state the word "So" on an in breath. On the next out breath, exhale the syllable "Ham." This is one cycle.

❸ Repeat the sounds on the in and out breaths, settling into a rhythm and working up to twelve cycles at first. Build up to twenty minutes over time, gradually making the iteration silent and the breath effortless.

❹ When you feel fully confident with the technique, start to use it silently in every situation during the day—waiting for a train, sitting in a dull meeting, playing sports. You will plant yourself in the present and link in with the inhalation and exhalation of the earth.

# don't panic

When you feel yourself hyperventilating—or unconsciously holding your breath—in the face of stress, focus yourself with this alternate-nostril breathing technique. You'll be concentrating so fully on following the instructions correctly that the stress has to take a backseat.

## anuloma viloma

❶ Sit comfortably upright. Fold the first and middle fingers on your right hand into your palm in Chin Mudra. Take your hand to your nose. Place the ring and little fingers on your left nostril, the thumb on your right nostril. Join the left thumb and first finger—Jnana Mudra.

❷ Close your eyes. Inhale through both nostrils, block your left nostril with the ring and little fingers, and exhale through your right nostril. Inhale though your right nostril, envisaging activating energy.

❸ At the top of the inhalation, block your right nostril with the thumb and exhale through your left nostril. Inhale through your left nostril, feeling a cooling detoxifying. This is one cycle. Repeat up to seven cycles. Finish on an exhalation from the right nostril, then inhale through both nostrils.

# mantra meditation

- **Chanting "Om"**
- **Using seed mantras**
- **Om mani padme hum**

Repeating a word or phrase over and over provides another focus to keep the mind from wandering. As you chant the mantra, your breathing becomes slower and more rhythmic, your mind fixes on the utterance, and the repetition stills and centers you. When the word repeated has significance, it starts to work on your consciousness so that your mind resonates with the meaning, changing the way you think. Think of it as resetting your default. Medical studies show that chanting lowers blood pressure, slows the heart rate, and boosts alpha brain waves (page 15) to charge you with energy. Mantras are considered powerful on a more subtle level, too, because they activate the energy of sound. When you chant, you create sound waves that resonate at certain frequencies. Many people believe that these intense vibrations empower, heal, cleanse away impurities, and revitalize different parts of the body as well as aspects of the mind and spirit. Once the mind has been emptied through meditation, it can be filled through repetition with the energy incarnate in the word.

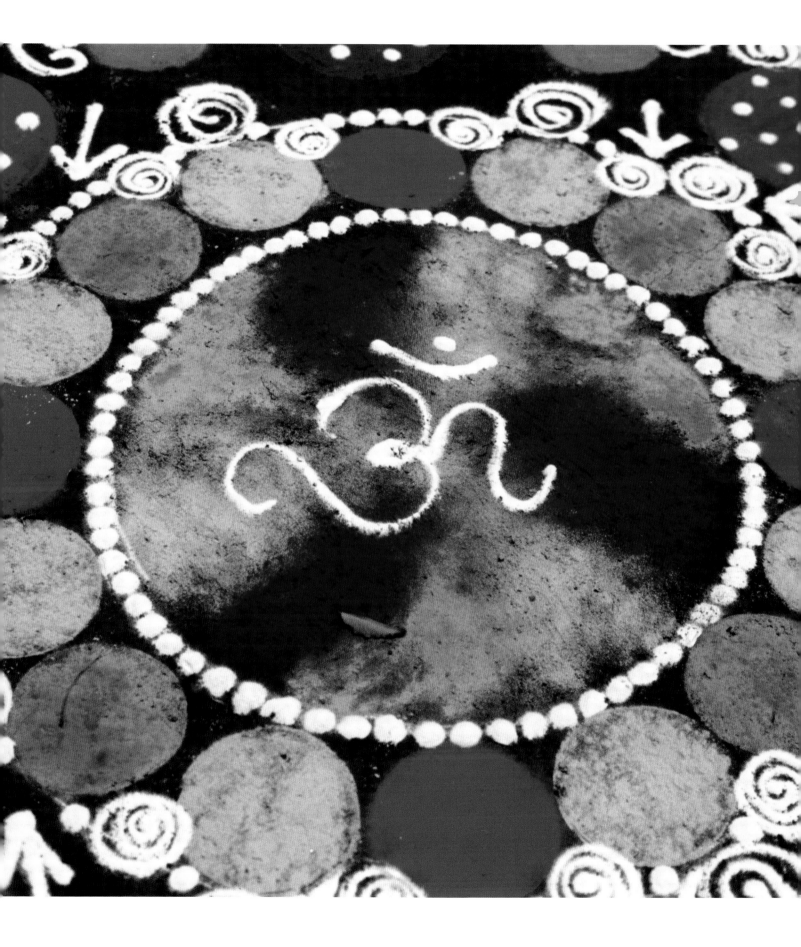

# chanting "om"

Composed of three sounds—A, U, M—the mantra "Om" is the most powerful there is, considered by Hindus and Buddhists to be the sound of the universe and the source of everything. The vibrations set up in its chanting are said to have brought all matter into being, and uttering it has a similarly transformative effect on the human body. As you yoke your breathing to the sound waves, the body's subtle energy centers clear, allowing vitality to flow unhindered through the body and illuminate the mind. Work toward making the sound silent, its most potent form. This chant is considered especially beneficial for men.

❶ Sit in a comfortable upright position, preferably in the Lotus or Half-lotus Pose (pages 22–23). Rest your hands on top of each other in your lap, palms up, thumb tips touching in Jnana Mudra (pages 26–27). Close your eyes and focus on the point between your eyebrows.

❷ Tune in to your breath for a few minutes, feeling your breathing deepen and lengthen as mind and body start to slow down.

❸ Take a deep in breath, feeling your diaphragm drop. Exhale the out breath with an open mouth, making the sound "Ahhh."

❹ As the breath hits your throat, turn it into an "Oooo" sound, letting it reverberate up from your solar plexus to your palate. Close your lips and feel it echo up into your head.

❺ Allow the sound to well up, vibrating in the crown of your head and in every part of your body, then escape through your lips in a prolonged "Mmmm." Let the sound drift away and don't hurry the next in breath: appreciate the silence and emptiness that follow the declaration.

❻ Let the in breath come naturally, then repeat the "Ahhh," "Oooo," and "Mmmm" sounds in the same way. When your mind wanders, bring it back to the sounds and your breath and try to melt into it, drawing inward and simultaneously sending the good vibes outward.

## finding your own mantra

Be your own teacher by selecting a personal mantra: try out any word or phrase that speaks to you, such as "peace," "love," "now," or "one," and play with it for a while. If it's not working, try another. You might find your mantra in the words of a song, ads on signs that you can't forget, or a bumper sticker that you see frequently. We are thought to be attracted to mantras that set up vibrations that the body can respond to: keep yourself open to all possibilities and you'll find something that works for you.

**left:** The auspicious Om symbol is ubiquitous in India; here it forms the center of a rangoli pattern made in colored powder.

# using seed mantras

Different energy centers in the body—chakras—respond to certain sound vibrations. When you chant these sounds, the subtle body resonates, retuning itself so energy can circulate freely, restoring you to total well-being. These sounds are referred to as "seeds"—*biji*—and are the source of power and meaning in a mantra, forming the building blocks of longer mantras. When you feel lackluster and out of sorts, try meditating on the chakras by chanting their seed sounds to bring harmony and well-being to every part of your life.

### crown chakra (crown of the head) *om*
Chanting brings about knowledge and heightened perception and deepens consciousness.

### root third eye chakra (between the eyes) *ksham*
Chanting calms the mind, reduces cravings, and can help with levels of concentration.

### base of the throat chakra (thyroid) *ham*
Brings you into harmony with the energy of ether and sense of hearing; chanting boosts communication and peace of mind; energizes the respiratory system.

### heart chakra (center of the chest) *yam*
Corresponds to air and the sense of touch; chanting evokes energy and enthusiasm; helps banish fear and grief; aids the circulatory system.

### navel chakra (solar plexus) *ram*
Stimulates fire energy and the sense of sight; chanting boosts willpower and motivation and works on the digestive system.

### pelvic chakra (deep in the pelvis) *vam*
Connects with water and taste sensations; chanting brings creativity and reduces pride; it boosts the urinary system and sexuality.

### root chakra (base of spine) *lam*
Correlates with the earth and sense of smell; chanting brings calmness and contentment and strengthens the excretory system.

❶ Before starting to meditate, choose a mantra that seems appropriate to your current situation: you might want to boost your creativity, alleviate a stomachache, or regain a zest for life, for instance. Memorize the sound.

❷ Sit with legs crossed and hands in Jnana Mudra (pages 22–27). Close your eyes and start to listen to your breathing for a few minutes.

❸ When you feel calm and centered, take a full, deep breath and start to chant the mantra on the out breath. With each exhalation repeat the sound, taking your focus to the part of the body it is associated with. Feel the vibration of the sound igniting a warmth and light in that part of the body. See this ball of light glowing with each repetition of the chant.

❹ You might also use an image of the associated element—earth, fire, water, air—to illuminate the chanting. Visualize the image as you repeat the mantra, fusing the sound and image into one entity.

❺ Work for three to five minutes, then just sit quietly as your body adjusts to the reverberations. If you prefer, lie back in the Corpse Pose, Savasana (pages 28–29), for a few minutes.

### seed sounds
By chanting these sounds you fuse yourself with the energies of the natural elements and enliven associated chakra energy centers, strengthening the body systems they govern.

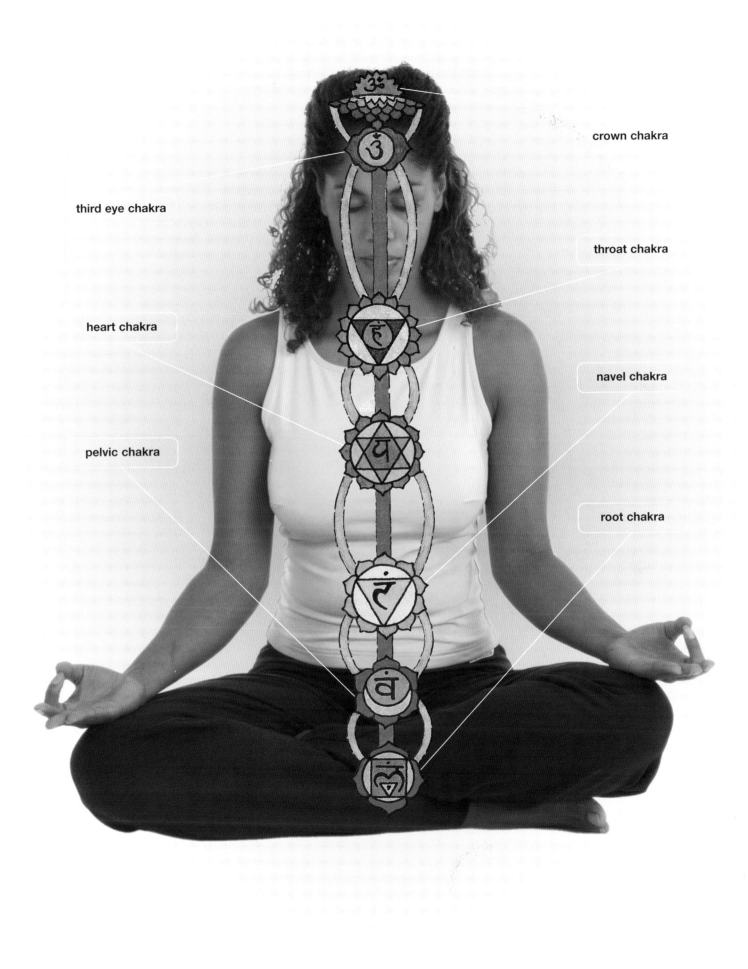

crown chakra

third eye chakra

throat chakra

heart chakra

navel chakra

pelvic chakra

root chakra

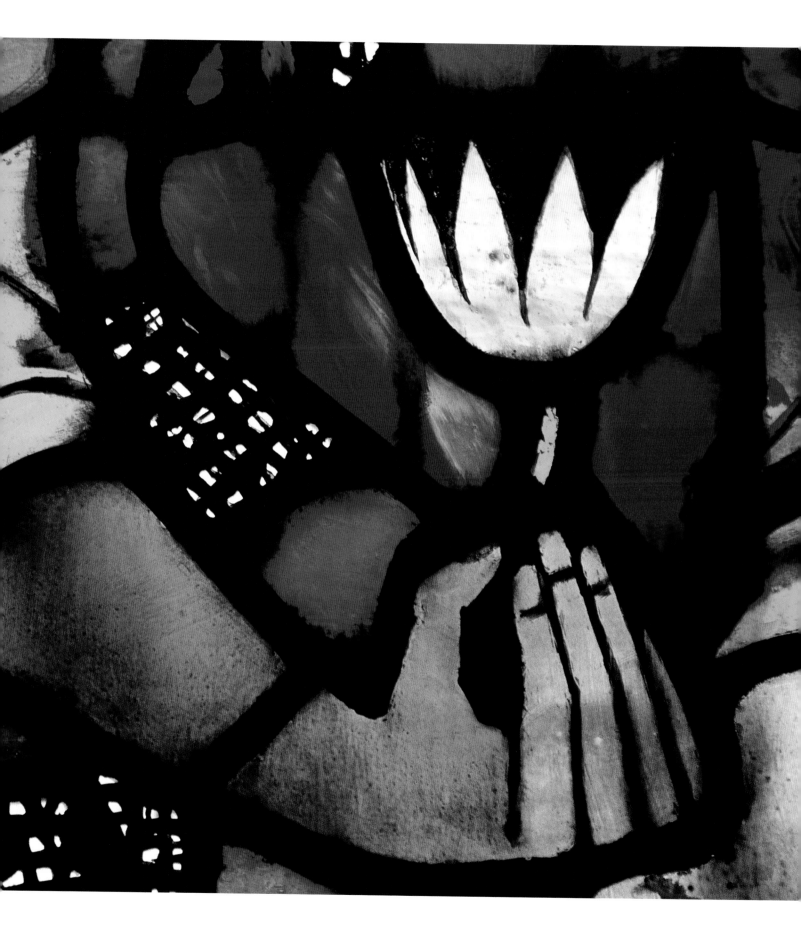

# om mani padme hum

This Tibetan Buddhist invocation offers another route into chanting meditation. Even non-Buddhists find the chanting over and over of a changing phrase helpful in lifting the mind away from preoccupations and calming the body. The transformative effect is embodied in the words, which translate as "Oh thou jewel in the lotus, hail!" Be inspired by the lotus, symbol of the potential of mankind with its roots in mud and fabulous bloom in sunlight. Contemplate, too, the light-reflecting purity of the precious jewel (representing the Buddha) shining out from the flower. Start this chant out loud, linking it in with your inhalations and exhalations like a breath meditation. When you feel at home with it, start to work silently.

❶ Sit comfortably upright, preferably in the Lotus or Half-lotus Pose (pages 22–23). Place the backs of your hands on your knees, palms relaxed, linking the tips of your thumbs and index fingers in Jnana Mudra (pages 26–27).

❷ Gently close your eyes and take your focus inside. Start to watch your breath, feeling it deep within your abdomen and allowing each in breath to come naturally.

❸ Inhale deeply and start to recite the words of the mantra out loud on the next exhalation; make the words fill the entire exhalation. Let the inhalation come easily; repeat the phrase on the next exhalation.

❹ As you chant, bring your focus to each of the six syllables in turn. When your mind wanders, bring it back to the anchor of these sounds.

❺ When the chant becomes familiar, visualize each of the syllables as the turning spokes of a wheel of light, generating energy as it rotates. See a protective energy shield surround you and absorb its light as you chant.

❻ After a while, start to project that same transforming light and energy back out to the universe. After you finish chanting, half-open your eyes, taking care to retain awareness of the light and energy within, and take this with you back into the world.

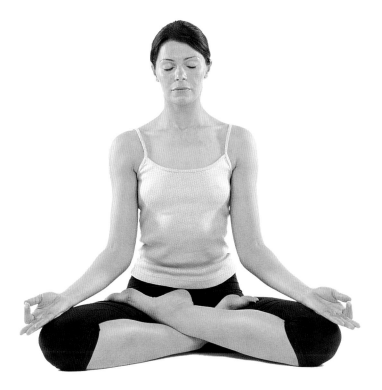

## lifting the spirit

Thankless physical tasks lend themselves well to mantra practice. Washing the car, chores such as painting walls or tiling, and even vacuuming take on greater significance when underpinned by the repetition of a mantra. With each tap of the hammer or stroke of the sponge, say the mantra, then when your mind wanders, the rhythmic actions bring you back to the word. Soon enough, you will find the mantra starts repeating itself, like a word from a seductive song, without you needing to initiate anything.

"The world is so constructed, that if you wish to enjoy its pleasures, you must also endure its pains."

**Swami Brahmananda**

# meditation for healing

- **Pain-relief visualization**
- **Distance healing**
- **Light visualization**

The mind can help the body heal. A considerable amount of research evidence attests to this, citing the placebo effect (when subjects respond to a course of "drugs" that were nothing more than sugar pills) as proof of the power of the mind to influence the body. Many meditative traditions use visualization techniques to involve people in the healing process. Ayurveda, for example, values meditation for its detoxing effect on mind and body, and for bringing together the head and the heart to share in healing. Increasingly in the West, family doctors and pain clinics refer patients with chronic pain to meditation sessions to learn relaxation and stress-relief techniques that can lessen the severity and even the frequency of symptoms. Simply relaxing the muscles is a very effective way to reduce the sensation of pain. Controversially, a number of research studies also report the healing effects of meditating or praying for others, even at a distance. Whether you are confronting surgery, have a chronic health condition, or simply suffer occasional mind-numbing headaches, what's sure is that staying positive and aware by investing yourself in the healing process through meditation will help you get better faster.

# pain-relief visualization

When faced with pain, it can be empowering to think positive using meditation techniques. Studies reveal that patients with chronic pain who practice mind-relaxation techniques report fewer symptoms of pain and psychological distress and visit the doctor less frequently. Before you start this meditative exercise, take a look at an anatomy book to familiarize yourself with the placement of the internal organs. Ask your doctor to explain what's going on in your body so you can adapt the techniques to reflect the healing process for your condition. With asthma, for example, you might envisage the bronchioles clearing and expanding to allow in fresh oxygen. Let meditation improve your quality of life.

❶ Sit or lie comfortably (pages 22–29). Close your eyes and take a few minutes to center yourself by witnessing the flow of breath in and out. When your mind wanders, keep bringing it back to the breath.

❷ Visualize your body as a whole: take your focus to the tips of your fingers, each shaft of hair, and your toenails. Scan the exterior of your body with your mind's eye.

❸ Now take your gaze inside. Visualize your internal organs: your heart and lungs, your kidneys and liver, your brain. Then imagine your veins and the blood coursing through them.

❹ Think about the pain and its site. See it as a color and shape, but keep it at a distance; don't let it engulf you and don't engage with it.

❺ Switch away from the area of pain and look at other parts of the body. If you have a headache, for example, think about your toes. Feel how mobile and free they are. There is no pain there. Move through the body, examining all the corners, seeing how little pain there is in these places.

❻ Having established how most of your body is not in pain, return to the site of the pain. Visualize the pain as an ice cube. With each out breath, take warmth and healing energy to the block of ice and, as if breathing on it, start to melt it. Little by little, visualize the warmth and your own healing energy reducing the size of the ice as the rest of your body enjoys its pain-free state.

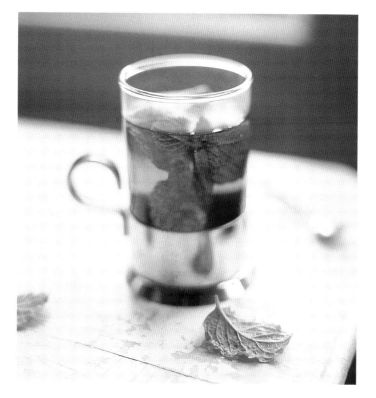

### healing mantra

Chanting the mantra "Sham" is thought in Ayurveda to help ease pain and reduce fever. As you chant, feel the essence of the sound filling up and empowering every cell.

### chakra visualization

Give the immune system a tune-up when you are feeling under the weather with the chakra visualization exercise on pages 120–21. Contemplate all the chakras in turn, working up from the root chakra. With each one, visualize healing energy brightening and lifting the energy center. Chant the sounds as you work if you like.

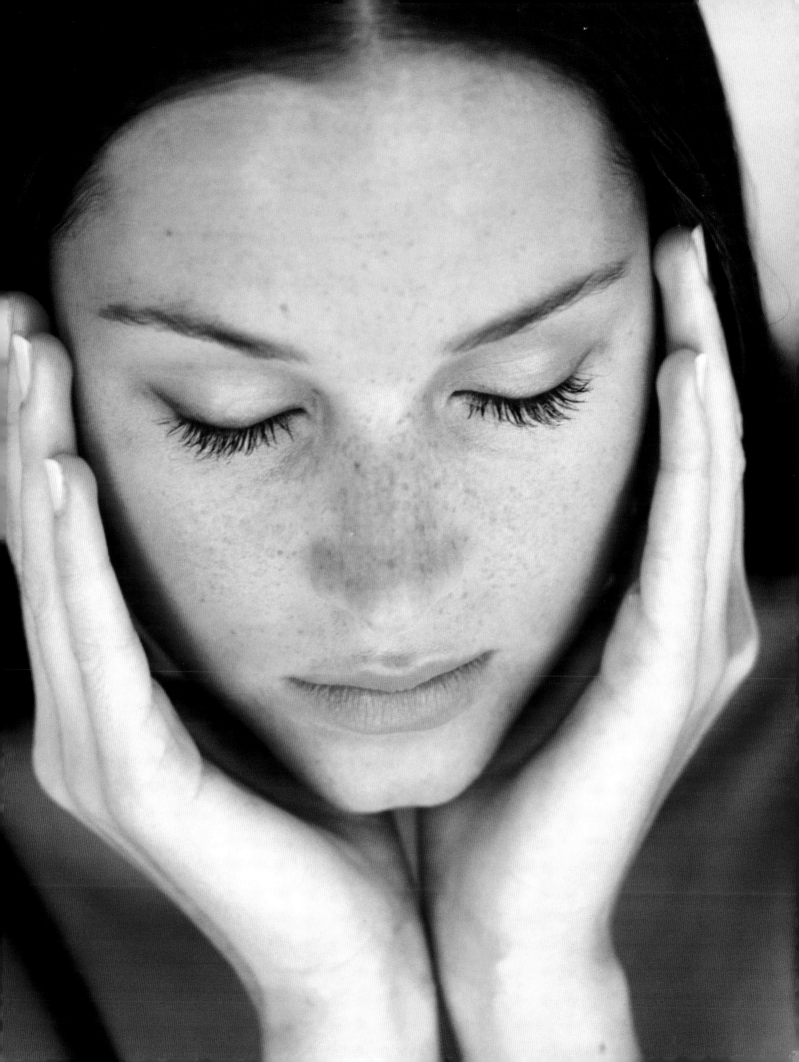

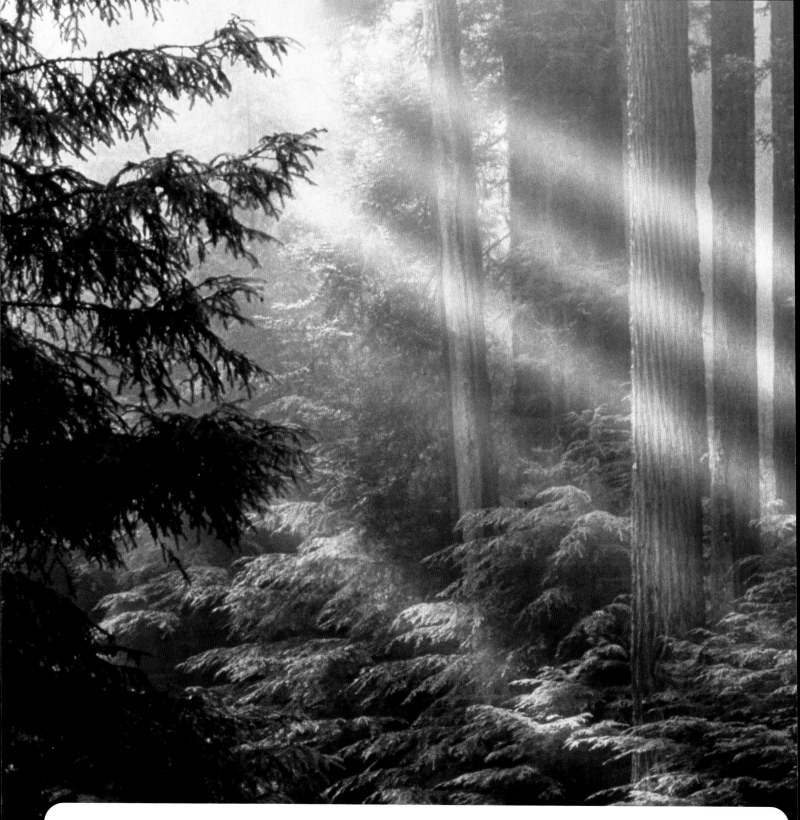

"I don't know if it helped him get better, but when I prayed for my grandpa to pull through his operation it made me feel more hopeful and able to cope."

Julia, secretary

# distance healing

Believe it or not, scientific research studies show that people who are prayed for when in ill health—animals and plants too—recover more often and more speedily than those who are not. In this exercise you send out vibes to aid self-healing. When you feel helpless and can do nothing else to help, at least you can do this, whether you are convinced by the evidence or remain skeptical.

❶ Sit or kneel comfortably upright (pages 22–25), bringing the hands together in one of the mudra hand gestures (pages 26–27).

❷ Feel your pelvis solid and centered down toward the earth. Pull up out of the pelvis, extending the spine to reach up to the sky. Sense the energy of the earth grounding you, and breathe in the energy of the ether.

❸ Close your eyes and focus on nothing but your breathing. For a few minutes become engrossed in the flow of air in and out.

❹ Focus your thoughts on the person you wish to help. To send your healing energy, you might want to pray for him or her if this feels right for you. Alternatively, visualize a healing light emanating from your heart. Let light, positivity, and hope well up; connect with this healing energy, then send it out to the person you wish to help. Imagine the light engulfing the recipient with warmth and healing energy. Visualize the person fit and well.

❺ Sit quietly for a while before opening your eyes and coming to. Work as often as you feel might be helpful.

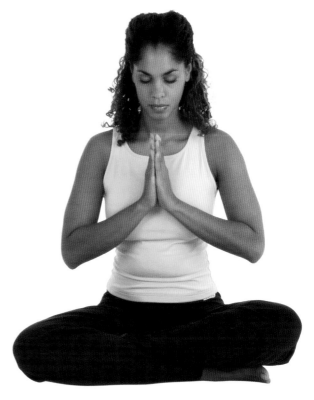

## healing chants

You might like to try chanting the traditional Indian mantra "Hari Om" for healing sick people who are far from you.

## fighting a virus

When you suffer from a virus there's little you can do except rest up and take lots of fluids. Antibiotics don't help, but this visualization might. Take your mind to the invader virus. Imagine the cells in your body. Now visualize your body's defense—white blood cells—coming to the rescue. See them enveloping the invaders and neutralizing their power. Imagine a cloak of whiteness overpowering inflamed viruses and destroying them.

Visualize these neutralized invaders being flushed out of your body through your nose when you blow it; spit them out when you need to. Simultaneously, visualize your body healing itself, with healthy cells regrouping to rebuild damaged structures. See every part becoming perfectly healthy. Imagine your limbs bursting with energy, feel your brain recharging, and let the whole body link together in perfect health.

# light visualization

This cleansing healing technique draws on the theory of color healing. Color healers teach that the vibrations of color waves purify and energize the invisible chakra energy centers that take in, process, and send energy around the body. By visualizing different frequency colors, you correct energy imbalances and create a state of balance and well-being. Certainly colors affect mood: bathing in red light boosts the heart rate and blood pressure; blue light decreases them. Even if you can't bring yourself to believe in color therapy, use this meditative method to boost your concentration while you bathe in healing light.

❶ Lie on your back, legs and arms outstretched in the yoga Corpse Pose, Savasana (pages 28–29). Close your eyes. Take a few minutes to relax every part of your body from the toes up. Connect with your reason for wanting to meditate today. Then focus on your breathing, sensing the inhalations and exhalations becoming longer and deeper.

❷ Imagine a ball of translucent light beneath your toes. Feel its clarity, purity, and cleansing energy. Bring the ball of light up to the base of your spine. Imagine it igniting a spark there and wiping out negativity.

❸ Take the ball of light to your pelvic region. Let it infuse this area with cleansing energy, light, and good health. Feel tension and anxiety dissolving. Move the ball of light up to your solar plexus and suffuse the whole of this region with well-being and goodness.

❹ Shift the ball of light into your heart area, where it brings nourishing positivity and vitality. Move it up to your throat. Feel the light washing away impurities, then bathe the region in empowering light and energy.

❺ Take the ball of light to the area between your eyebrows. Feel it dissolving physical and mental blocks and igniting the area with healing light. Move the ball of light to hover just above the crown of your head. See it turn with energy, sending out vibrations of intense light and goodness.

❻ Finally, let a ray of radiant, life-giving light join all the energy centers you have spotlighted to create a straight line from toe to head. Sense the liberation of enlightenment.

❼ When you have time, repeat the exercise, visualizing balls of light colored red, orange, yellow, green, blue, indigo, and violet. Breathe in the colors, letting each tone in the spectrum fill you with its own unique energy.

"I wear orange when I'm feeling down and imagine myself taking a shower of orange light. My coworkers think I'm nuts, but it keeps me happy and outgoing."

Gabriela, bank clerk

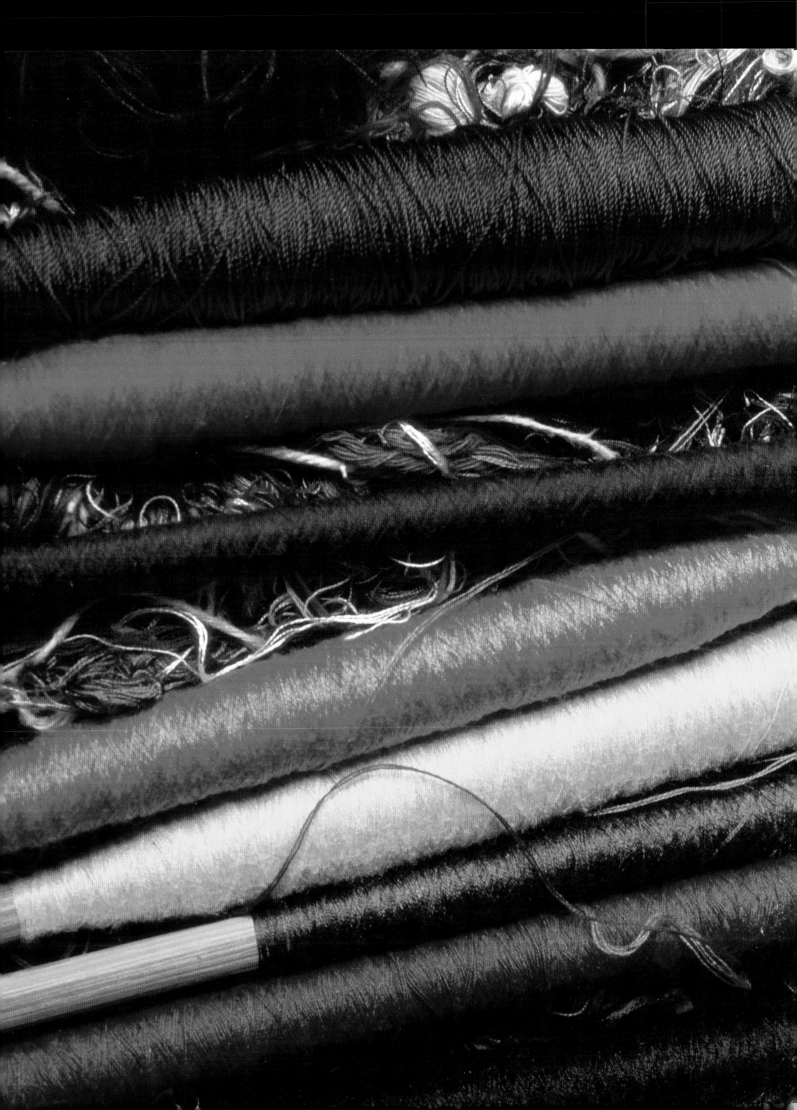

"We are what we think. All that we are arises with our thoughts."

**The Buddha**

# self-help meditation

- **Getting to know yourself**
- **Widening your horizons**
- **Becoming patient**
- **Forgiving yourself**
- **Managing anger**

When you start to meditate it can feel like closing in on yourself and keeping the world outside at arm's length. As you work with the techniques, you start to notice in greater detail how you respond to your unique flow of thoughts and to interruptions from outside. You get to watch your mind pulling you this way and that as thoughts intrude into your practice. In this way, meditation teaches you about what makes you tick—your emotions and how you mediate them, your take on the world, what you're happy with, and what you'd like to change. The meditations that follow help you explore the complexity of your personality and understand what keeps you from relaxing fully: perhaps a lack of patience, good humor, or peace of mind. At its core, meditation boosts your happiness by steering you toward ways of acting that make you more confident, complete, vital, and ready to interact with others.

# getting to know yourself

Through meditation you get to see how changeable the mind is. Ask it to be still for even a minute, and it can't. As you watch it wandering, you realize that the mind doesn't define who you are. When you work with sense meditations (pages 58–79), you start to appreciate the array of ever-changing sensations that the body and mind experience. This, then, is not you either. The body is constantly evolving, too. This is most obvious in childhood and adolescence, but as adults we also see the changes daily: new wrinkles, extra folds of skin, weight lost and put back on again. And as cells die and new cells are created, the body is always in a state of turnover—no part of the body remains constant. What is constant? This meditation helps you explore the core within that makes you what you are. It also gives you the empowering knowledge that you are in charge, free to do with your awareness what you will.

❶ Sit or kneel in a comfortable upright position, hands resting on knees or thighs (pages 22–27). Close your eyes. Take a few moments to calm and focus your mind by watching the waves of breath moving in and out.

❷ When your mind feels tranquil, start to ponder your body. Imagine your fingers and toes when you were a newborn baby; visualize your arms and legs as a two-year-old and six-year-old; think about the changes of adolescence; imagine your brain and kidneys when you were a fetus; picture your hair and your spine when you are older; if you are a woman, imagine or remember the physical changes of pregnancy. Understand that the body is constantly in flux, that it does not define who you are.

❸ Start to watch your mind. See it as a blank screen, then without engaging with them, watch thoughts projected onto it. See how you remain separate from your thoughts. They are not you.

❹ Now notice sensations: pins and needles in your legs, perhaps, an itchy nose, an urge to sneeze, sounds beyond the room, and the air on bare skin. See how the sensations change as you let time pass, and understand that stimulation of the sense receptors is separate from you.

❺ Appreciate the freedom of not having to be your thoughts, emotions, body, or sensations. Relish the potential this represents. Make the choice now to use this knowledge next time you are carried away by anger or overexcitement, by peer pressure or the urge to consume. Use this knowledge to help you decide what you want from life and to make the changes and take action to bring it about.

# sky bathing

Tibetan monks and nuns lie on their backs and stare out into the blue, cloudless sky as a meditation exercise. Try it yourself to gain a sense of spaciousness and appreciation of the possibilities life offers; allow gazing into space to widen your horizons.

"Utterly exhausted from climbing 4,000 feet, I look out, watching the rain clouds head in, and get that wonderful feeling that I don't matter."

Ben, climber

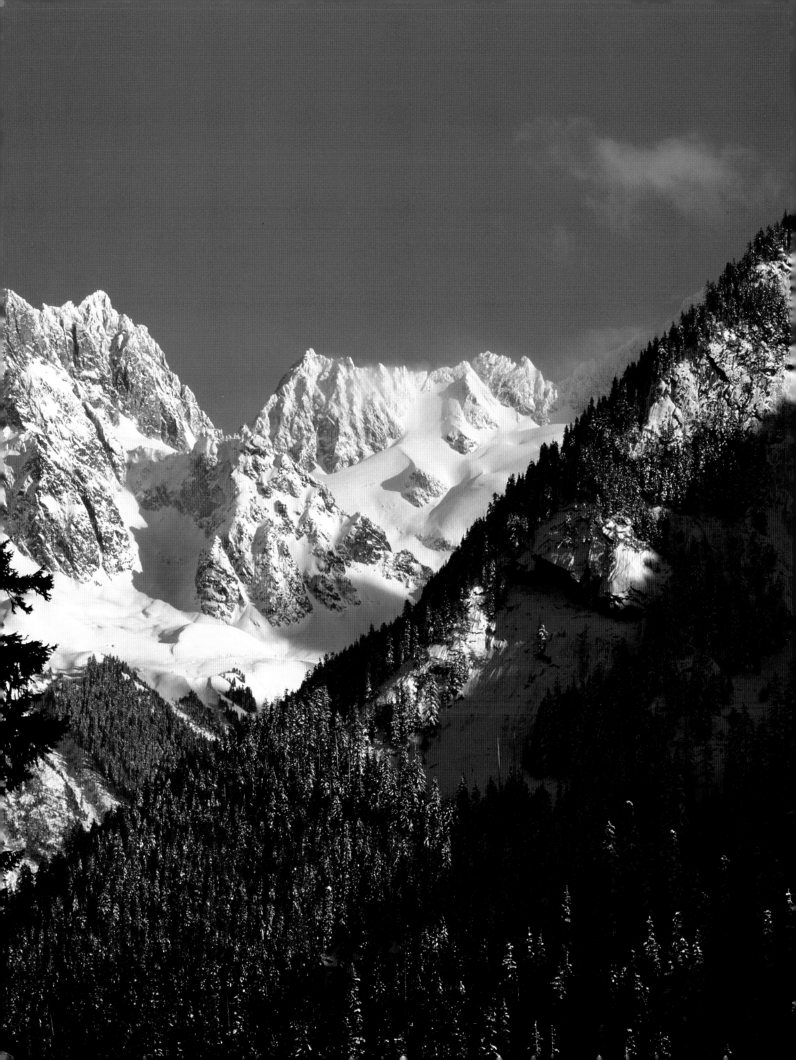

# widening your horizons

Spaciousness is a state of mind you can cultivate through meditation. This quality enables you to step away from the habitual treadmill of work, eat, sleep, work that encourages self-limiting ways of thinking and behaving. Finding vastness of mind liberates you to think outside the box, to open up to all possibilities and potential. This can transform your career, your relationships, and your lifestyle by helping you find spontaneity, see the bigger picture, understand from other points of view, and above all maintain that youthful belief that life offers you infinite choices and everything is there for the taking.

❶ Sit comfortably upright, hands resting on knees or thighs (pages 22–27). Close your eyes. Bring yourself inside to focus on the movement of breath in and out. When thoughts or sensations intrude, simply acknowledge them and ask them to leave. Be patient.

❷ Imagine you are sitting on the edge of a cliff, on a hill overlooking a field, or on a wide beach looking out to the sea. In your mind's eye, watch the horizon: see how wide, distant, and open it is. Imagine looking up at the sky, feeling the vast dome arching from horizon to horizon. Sense its spaciousness. You may feel dizzy at the scale and expanse.

❸ When thoughts occur, visualize them appearing on the horizon, so far away that they no longer have any urgency. Let them slip below the horizon.

❹ If it helps, have someone read to you the quotation below, extracts from a scene in Shakespeare's *King Lear*, to conjure up an illusory clifftop to a blind man.

❺ Take the feeling of expanse and spaciousness within you. Visualize it expanding your internal organs, including your lungs and your brain.

❻ Bring yourself back to your body by sensing your sitting bones making contact with the ground. Take your focus to your breath and draw it downward. Feel the inhalation cause your abdomen to expand and the exhalation draw your abdomen toward your lower back. Breathe from beneath the earth, imagining it seeping up into your feet and buttocks to ground you. Sit quietly for a few minutes to remove any lasting sensations of dizziness.

"How fearful
And dizzy 'tis to cast one's eyes so low!
The crows and choughs that wing the midway air
Show scarce so gross as beetles . . .
The fishermen that walk upon the beach
Appear like mice . . .
The murmuring surge,
That on th' unnumbered idle pebble chafes,
Cannot be heard so high. I'll look no more,
Lest my brain turn, and the deficient sight
Topple down headlong."

*King Lear*, Act IV, Scene VI

# becoming patient

Meditation is hardest for those of us who can't stand to be still, those who can't wait and won't try. But it offers great results. When you feel angry, irritated, frustrated, or trapped, don't be hard on yourself, just switch off with this time-out meditation. It gives you a break that allows you to reflect on the effects such negativity has on you and others. Then try the Smile of the Buddha exercise to reset your responses into a tranquillity zone.

❶ When you just can't sit still or wait for something, go for a walk. First of all, focus on your pace and on your breath, watching how the in and out breaths come into coordination with the movement of your limbs.

❷ When you've relaxed, start to think about how impatience makes you feel. Don't get caught up on the minutiae of the subjects, just feel how it affects your body and mind.

❸ Next think about how your impatience affects others: those you work and live with; people you have to get along with even if you don't like being with them. Again, don't get caught up in the details.

❹ Switch your thoughts to how patience might solve the negativity your impatience creates. How much better might you feel? How much more positive might your interactions with others be? Become absorbed in the sensations of peace, cooperation, and happiness that this might bring. Try to return to these sensations throughout the day to start resetting your relationship with the world.

# the smile of the buddha

Look at a depiction of the Buddha and there's always a slight smile on the face that suggests patience, acceptance, and contentment as well as compassion, humility, and infinite grace. This exercise teaches how to take a smile within.

❶ Sit or kneel comfortably upright (pages 22–25), placing your hands in Cosmic Mudra (page 26). Close your eyes, relax the muscles in your face, and focus on your breathing.

❷ When you feel calm and untroubled, start smiling—not a clown's grimace, but a gentle upturn of the lips and face that extends subtly around to the ears and up to the temples. It can help to focus on the third eye area between your brows.

❸ Take the smile inside to diffuse throughout your body. First take it to your heart; imagine your heart smiling, strange as this sounds. As you breathe in, let the smile suffuse your lungs. Then take the smile out from your lungs with the oxygen and into your bloodstream. Let it light up every part that the blood reaches: little toes to elbows, thighs to throat. As you bring the smile to each area, feel your muscles relax and a sense of lightness lift the body.

❹ When the whole body is tingling with brightness, let the positive energy of the smile fill your brain; focus it between your eyes and let it extend up to the crown of your head.

❺ At the end of your meditation, half-open your eyes, retaining awareness of the lightness and smile within as you reenter the world.

**right:** The half-closed eyes of the Buddha—this statue is from the Po Lin Monastery in Hong Kong—reveal a state of deep meditation.

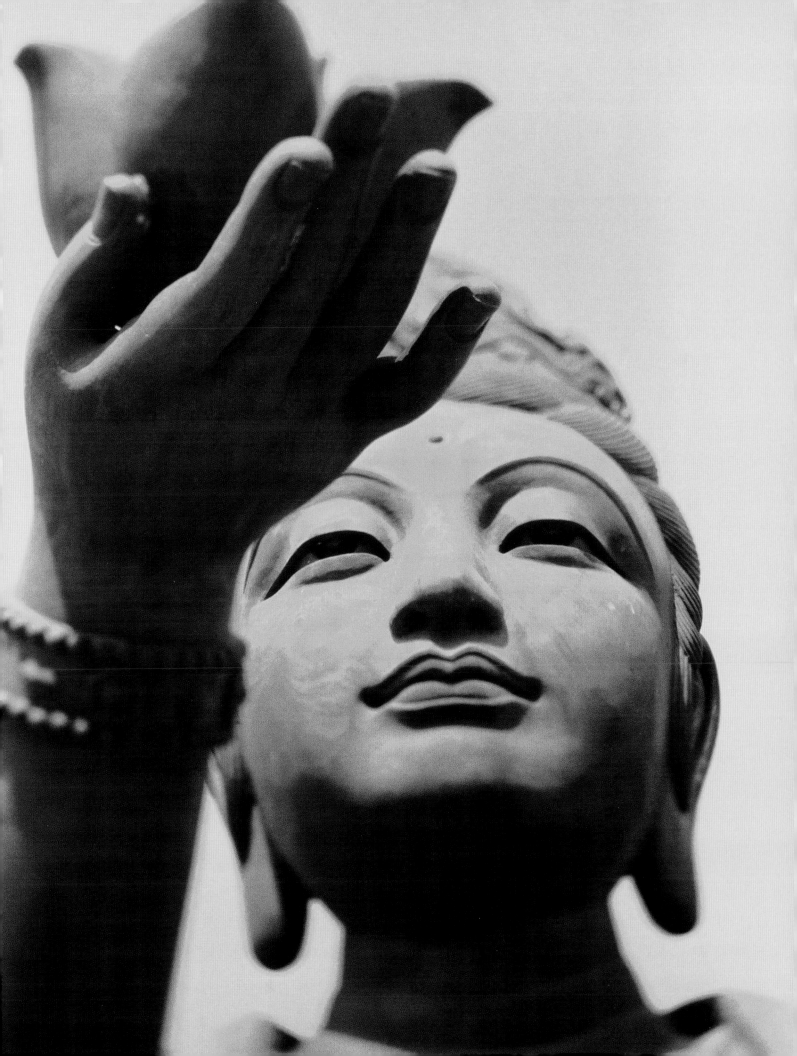

# forgiving yourself

Cell phones, e-mail, text messages, and deadlines mean we rarely get private time to relax and just be ourselves. A common reaction to the stresses and strains of modern living is to feel guilty, be it because you failed to meet an important deadline, finish all your work by the end of the day, forgot to send a birthday card, or didn't have time to go to the gym. Sahaja yoga is an easy-to-learn meditation technique that is very effective at assuaging the self-loathing that can result from these feelings of guilt. It works with kundalini, a nurturing or mothering energy within, using affirmations and hand movements gently to massage the chakra energy centers. You don't have to believe in the theory behind this technique, developed by Shri Mataji Nirmala Devi, to benefit from its effects. Just follow the steps to move effortlessly into the meditative state, integrating your head with your heart and letting go of your troubles.

❶ Sit in a comfortable upright position, hands resting on your knees or thighs (pages 22–24), palms up. Take a few moments to quiet your brain and focus inside.

❷ Place your right palm on your left side at the lower part of your abdomen. Address the nurturing energy within you, saying to yourself silently, "Mother, please awaken the pure knowledge in me." Repeat the statement six times.

❸ Move your palm to the upper part of your abdomen and state the empowering affirmation, "Mother, I am my own master." Repeat ten times.

❹ Place your right palm over your heart (on the left side of the chest) and use this affirmation, "Mother, I am the spirit." Repeat twelve times.

❺ Turn your head to look over your right shoulder and place your palm where your left shoulder meets your neck. Give it a squeeze. State to yourself sixteen times, "Mother, I feel no guilt at all." Say it with meaning.

❻ Place your palm over your forehead. Massage away any tension by squeezing at the temples, then repeat to yourself the following affirmation, "Mother, I forgive everyone and myself." Don't think of anyone in particular while you do this, just be sincere.

❼ Take your palm to the back of your head and ask yourself for forgiveness, saying, "Please forgive any mistakes I have made, knowingly or unknowingly." Don't wallow in guilt, just let it go.

❽ Place your palm on the crown of your head and massage the scalp, moving the skin in a clockwise direction seven times, stating each time, "Mother, please let me experience pure awareness."

❾ Raise your palm a few inches above the crown of your head and just sit. You may feel a cool breeze on your palm emanating from the fontanelle at the crown of the head. Bring your right hand down and sit quietly for a while before opening your eyes.

## forgiveness breathing

Try this quick technique when you feel overwhelmed with guilt, but don't have time for the Sahaja yoga meditation. As you inhale, picture forgiving energy filling every cell within your body, zapping fear and self-loathing. Hold the breath for a couple of seconds to maximize the cleansing effect. Start to exhale slowly, visualizing all the mental and emotional toxins being expelled with the carbon dioxide. Breathe out fully and hold the lungs empty very briefly. Imagine another cleansing breath filling you as you inhale, and repeat the exercise for as long as it takes to ease your disquiet.

# managing anger

Use meditation proactively to turn rage and other negative emotions into positive energy and spur you toward change. After a few weeks of practice you will reach the point at which the first stirrings of anger will enable you to see what's what. They give you insight into your own nature and the state of the world. You stop being complacent and self-satisfied and become determined to change and steer your life in a better direction. You stop fretting and start doing something about it. Instead of creating more suffering, you harness suffering and turn it into goodness, finding out that you are much more than the victim of circumstance.

❶ When you feel anger engulfing you, transcend your usual reactions to catch your ego at work. Challenge it by waking up to the effects it's having on you. Examine your heart rate; listen to your breathing. Stand outside yourself and take a good look at what you look like. What's happened to you?

❷ Broaden your awareness to see the consequences of the angry acts or words not only on your body, but on your place in society and on others who have to endure the emotion with you. Think about the people in the room, think about those who have to live with the idea of you as an angry, irrational person. Just trying to maintain this awareness diffuses the emotion and provides the motivation to make the change.

❸ Now picture yourself happy and relaxed. What's your body language now? How do you feel inside? Consciously try to become this vision of yourself. Radiate what you want to be. Don't just think about, but feel the beneficial consequences. Do this every time you feel the anger coming on, trying to identify the very moment the rage starts welling up.

## the big picture

It may sound perverse, but staying more positive may be a case of contemplating death every day. The dying English playwright Dennis Potter in his last few weeks spoke of seeing the blossom on trees outside his window as the "blossomest blossom." Indeed, it's only when jolted into awareness by the notion of leaving everything behind that we make the effort to appreciate life and get the most out of every minute. If you're confronted with severe illness or death, contemplate it seriously. Use the distance healing meditation (pages 128–29) if it helps. But don't wallow in the sadness. Use this jolt to make the decision to make your life better and to strive to ease the lives of all those you have contact with.

## finding the time

The common cry is, "I want to change, but I'm too busy to find the time." Don't let this be your excuse. If you really want to make a difference you'll find the time by prioritizing and rethinking your day. Grab lost minutes to work on meditation: daydreaming on the morning commute, walking the dog, or even sitting in the bathroom. To get over impatience, anger, and frustration, perform mindless tasks with mindfulness to cultivate broadened awareness. Use the spaciousness technique (page 137) for ten seconds before you speak out in anger. Meditation isn't just something you set aside an hour to do every day, like an aerobics class—it gets inside you to inform your every move and thought, eventually becoming effortless and timeless.

"He who knows others is wise, he who knows himself is enlightened."

**Lao Tzu**

# meditation for others

- **Meditating with a partner**
- **Developing compassion**
- **Loving-kindness meditation**
- **Meditation for peace**

Because meditation makes you a nicer person—more relaxed, open, and compassionate—one of its benefits is better relationships with friends, lovers, family, and the world in general. This doesn't have to mean meditating with other people, though meditating in a room with strangers can be surprisingly calming and energizing; it means trying out the techniques that follow to understand that you're a cog in a machine and that when you function well, so do all the other parts. After you have worked for a while on ridding yourself of anger and guilt and building patience and a wider world view by using the exercises in the previous chapter, start with the meditations that follow to develop empathy, compassion, love, and respect for others; in the end, only this will bring us world peace.

# meditating with a partner

When you begin meditating, the last thing you might contemplate is involving other people. But some of the best meditation is done with others—think of how, while making love, two people inhabit the present totally. This moving meditation based on partner yoga gets you thinking about how much you rely on other people. Use it to understand more about communication and trust, compromise and difference, cooperation and balance, manipulation and judgment. Let the knowledge you gain about how you work with a yoga partner inform the way you deal with other people.

❶ Sit back-to-back with your partner, legs crossed comfortably. Shuffle your sitting bones back until the bases of your spines meet, then extend out of your pelvis and pull your abdomen in and up, allowing your lower back to support your partner's spine. Lengthen your middle and upper back, releasing against the support of your partner. Tuck your chin in slightly to extend the back of the neck and let the backs of your heads rest against each other. Drop your shoulders down and away from your ears and broaden your chest so that your upper backs touch and support each other. Rest your hands, palms up, on your knees or thighs.

❷ Balance your weight against each other, giving and taking until you both feel comfortably supported by the other. Now concentrate on your breathing, feeling your shoulders drop with the exhalation and letting the inhalation come naturally to expand the abdomen and rib cage. Be aware of your partner's breathing pattern and try to link together your inhalations and exhalations. Work for three to five minutes.

❸ Stand up and face each other. Place your feet hip-width apart, a few inches from your partner's feet, and stand tall. Grasp arms by holding around each other's wrists. Carefully lean back until your arms are straight. Shift your weight so that neither one of you is pulling the other off balance. Relax backward without collapsing your chest and keep your pelvis lifting. Look at each other.

❹ Exhaling, slowly bend your knees and start to descend into a squat, as if you are both sitting back on imaginary chairs. Go at a pace that you both feel happy with, inching down until your thighs make a right angle with the floor. As you increase in confidence about your partner's support, lean back more: this makes the movement easier. Look at each other and hold for a few moments, breathing evenly. Inhale as you stand up together. Repeat a few times.

## partner breathing

To sharpen the special connection you have with a partner or child, every so often link your breathing patterns together. This can be effective after an argument or when you've spent time apart. Sit facing each other or lie down so your bodies touch. Take turns matching your flow of breath in and out with that of your partner, following the lead of his or her inhalations and exhalations. Don't rush or get annoyed with the speed of the other person's pattern; just be like him or her. As you inhale, breathe in what makes this person special; as you exhale, feel your bodies dissolving as you are united in the breath.

## "You are among your family."

**Bedouin greeting**

"Entering a room filled with silent strangers freaked me out at first. Now knowing I can just sit there with people I don't know without having to make small talk is such a relief."

**Lateesha, architect**

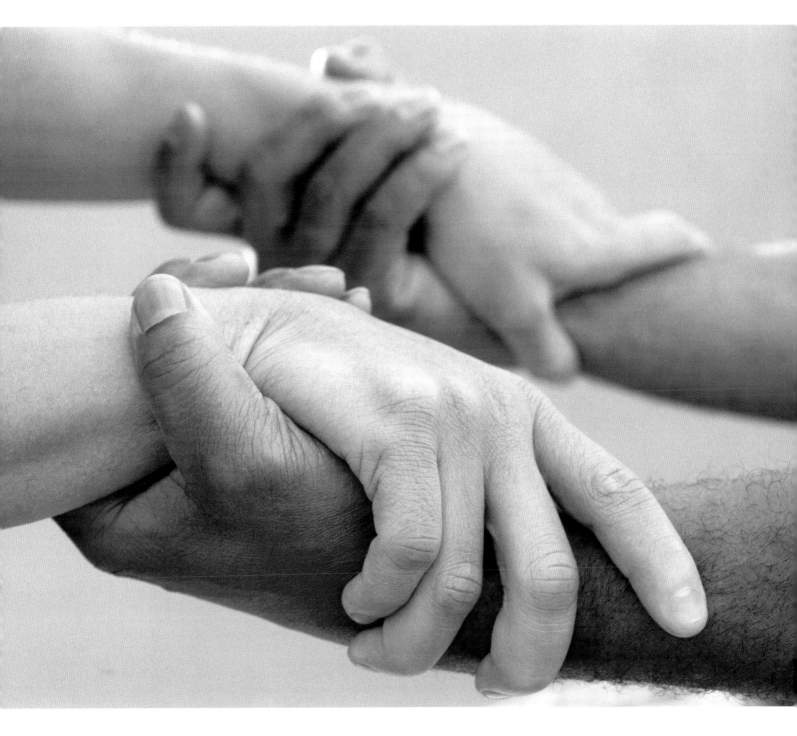

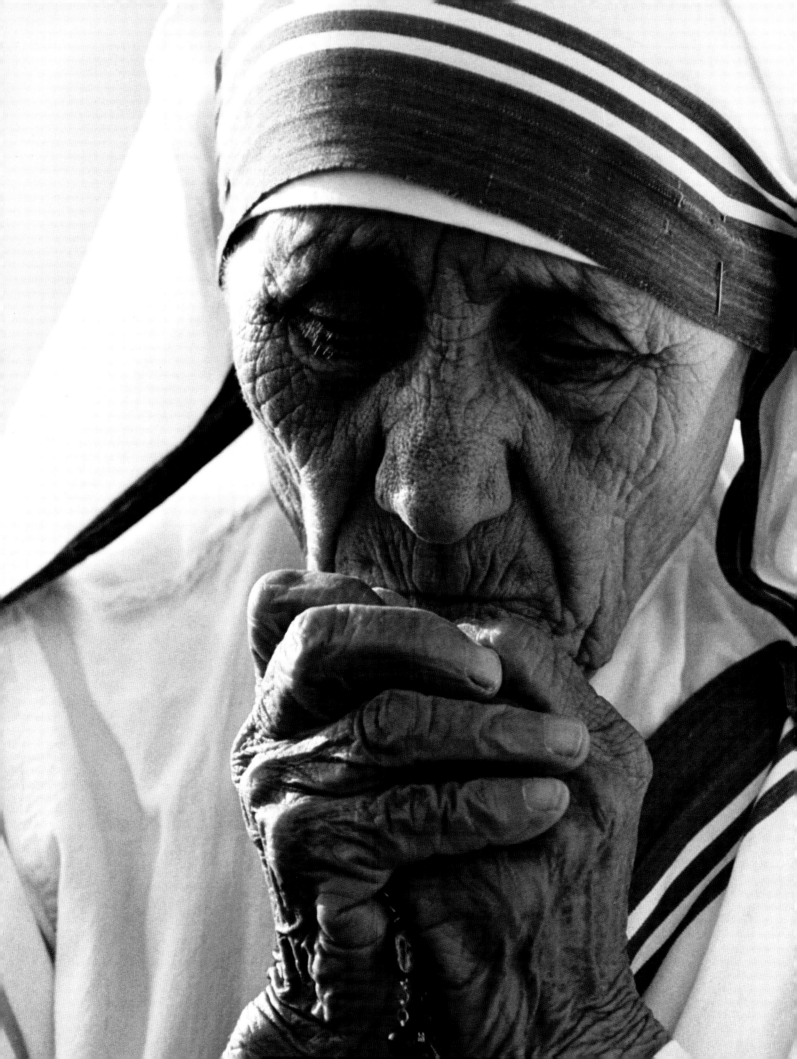

# developing compassion

It's human nature—survival of the fittest, one might say—to avoid actions and emotions that cause us suffering, and opt for things that make us feel good. This breathing exercise directly contradicts that. In the Tibetan Buddhist meditation known as *tonglen*, literally "giving and taking," you embrace pain and suffering, using the experience of badness to create some goodness—the cleansing away of selfishness and the awakening of your innate ability to empathize with others and show compassion. This can be life-affirming, and by contrasting your life with the lives of others, can also inspire thankfulness, appreciation of your lot, and encourage you to get out there and do something practical to relieve suffering around the world.

❶ Work sitting, standing, or moving, in a meditation space or outside. Whatever your situation, take a few moments to center yourself within and clear your thoughts, watching your breathing become calm and regular.

❷ When you feel ready, think about someone you know or people in the news who are suffering. On your next inhalation, try to suck in their pain and fear; take it on and make it your own. Visualize the breath as dark, cloudy, and heavy. If this feels too scary at first, inhale the wish to relieve the pain.

❸ As you exhale, send out compassion and understanding, love and healing, relaxation and happiness to relieve the suffering of the people you are thinking about. See the exhalation as a translucent, bright light.

❹ Work with this breathing pattern for a few minutes, imagining the inhalation drawing in through every pore and the exhalation flooding out through every pore.

## meditating on the street

You can make this meditation work in more practical circumstances, too. When you see people suffering physically or emotionally during your day, breathe it in as it's happening, feel and understand the pain, then exhale goodness, strength, healing, and light to neutralize the badness.

## compassion for you

You might find as you practice this technique that you recognize your own suffering in the pain of others. If so, stand back and repeat the exercise, working for yourself. Breathe in your pain and exhale relief from it. After a while, breathe in the pain of all those who are suffering the same sensation at this moment around the world. Let your heart absorb that suffering. Then breathe out love, release from suffering, understanding, and forgiveness to yourself and everyone else in the same situation right now. Expand it outward and see how large your compassion grows.

"We must give to each other until it hurts."

Mother Teresa

# loving-kindness meditation

This technique forms part of the de-stress armory of many people who practice yoga and meditation. In this Tibetan Buddhist practice known as *metta bhavana*, or "cultivating loving kindness," you start by enveloping yourself in loving kindness and then, bit by bit, work to send out this sensation to friends, strangers, enemies, and then the whole world. It develops your innate compassion, kindness, tolerance, and empathy. It shows you how to love yourself, a necessary precursor to reducing intolerance and hatred in the world. It also offers a way of connecting with the anonymous mass of people who you otherwise never get to reach—the strangers you pass every day on the street—which opens you up to be more humane in the way you treat people you have to interact with but don't know. Spend a discreet ten to fifteen minutes practicing each of the steps below before you move on to the next stage.

❶ Sit comfortably upright, hands resting on your knees or thighs (pages 22–25). Close your eyes and take your focus inside, watching your breathing slow and lengthen as you become more relaxed. Take your focus to your heart region and look at how you feel right now, without analyzing it or getting lost in thoughts. Smile and notice how this lifts you. After a while, bring your attention back to your breathing.

❷ Now remember a time at which you felt good about yourself: maybe you just got a promotion, became a parent for the first time, or were surrounded by friends. Conjure up the scents and sounds of that time, remember what you were wearing and where you were. All this helps you reinhabit these idyllic emotions. Let the sensations of happiness, security, and inner peace flood through you, and revel in your positive qualities.

❸ Link these feelings with the following phrase by repeating it slowly and silently on three exhalations: "May I be perfectly happy, may I be well, may I be free from pain." Inhale between each part of the phrase, watching how it makes you feel. If you prefer, make up your own words to express the same desires. Spend ten to fifteen minutes working up to this stage at first; you may want to do this for some weeks until you feel ready to move on.

❹ Think about someone who you know well and like—a good friend. See the person in your mind's eye if it helps, or remember a time you enjoyed together. Let the feeling of love and security you conjured up in step 2 fill your heart. Then send out those feelings, imagining them enveloping that person. Say the phrase, "May he be perfectly happy, may he be well, may he be free from pain."

❺ When you feel ready to do so, think about someone you don't know well but who you might see every day as you go about your daily routines: the person who serves your coffee or sells you the newspaper, the person who sometimes sits next to you on the bus. Call up those same feelings again; this time, extend them to this person. Repeat the phrases you used in step 4. Switch off your neutrality and imagine the recipient enveloped in security and unconditional love.

❻ Now think of someone you actively dislike, someone who may have caused you pain. Look at the feelings that arise in you when you think about that person. Try to think about that person's good side and about how much happier you could both be if you let go of your negativity. See that you have a choice and don't necessarily have to follow where your feelings lead. Now conjure up your happiness scene and let those feelings of love and security erase the uncomfortable feelings that may have been holding you back for some time now. Without thinking too much, send this love out to your enemy, repeating the phrases. Include yourself, too, if it helps, saying, "May we be perfectly happy." Let this color the way you react to that person the next time you see him. Smile, perhaps, and see over time the difference you can make.

❼ Finally, bring up the feelings of happiness and peace, then radiate them out to every person—every sentient animal, too—in the world. Start with your house, block, street, city, state, country, continent, until you've spread the net of well-wishing as wide as it will possibly stretch. After finishing, sit quietly for a while with your body relaxed as you adjust to being back in the room.

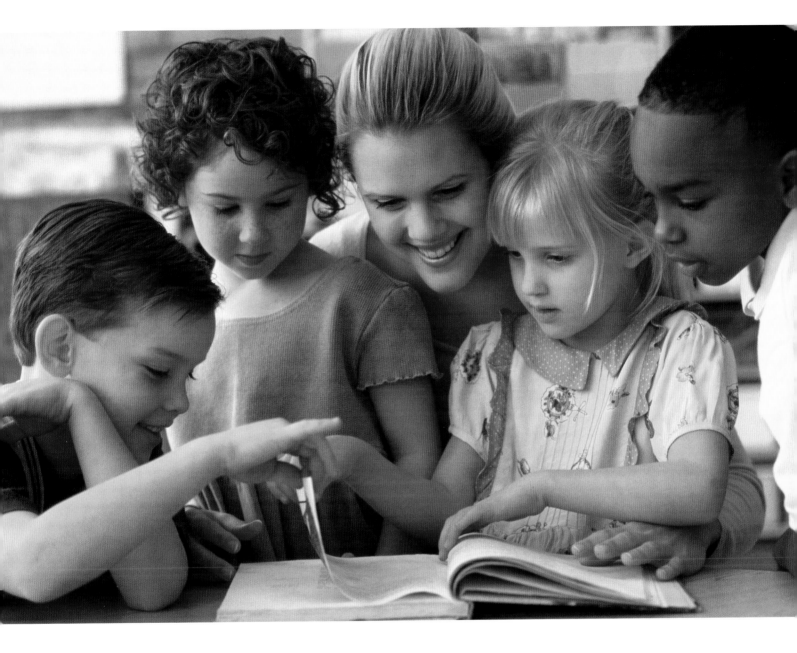

## concrete meditation

Put your meditation into action by doing some good in your own community. Offer to read for young children, become a mentor for teenagers, volunteer at a project for homeless people, befriend an elderly neighbor, or find some other charity work to make concrete the aims you have nurtured with meditation.

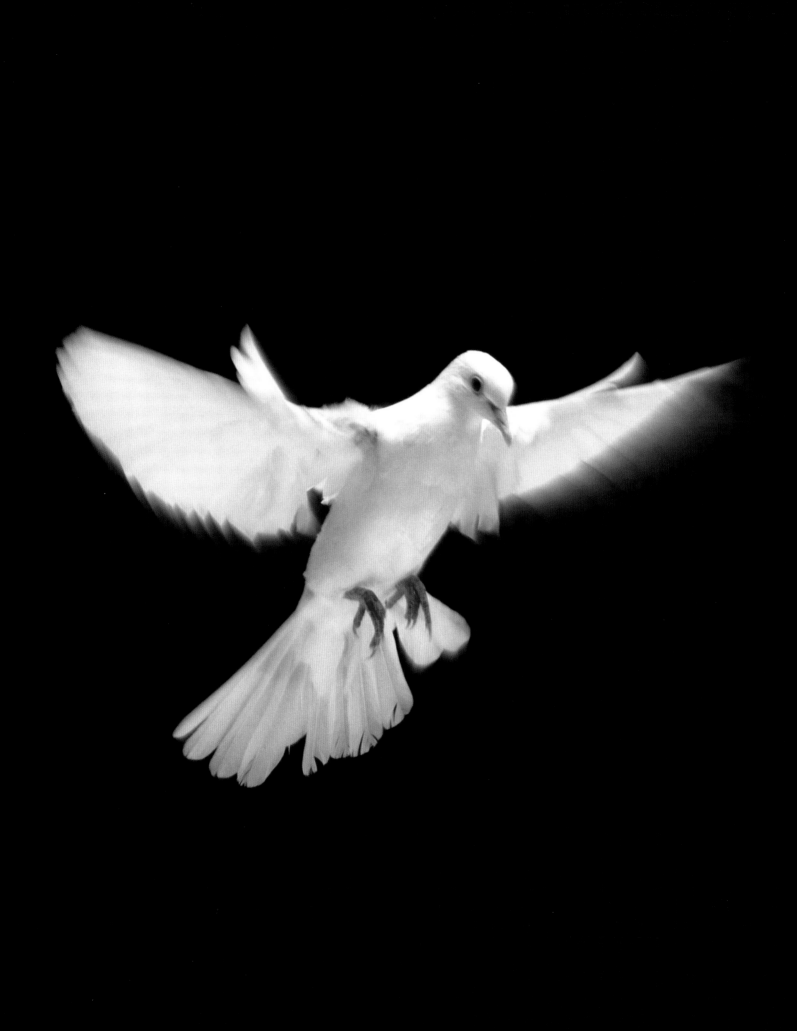

# meditation for peace

What we're all really searching for is peace. When you're trying to find inner peace, it makes sense to mirror your work with an active exploration of ways to increase the peace worldwide.

❶ Sit comfortably upright, hands resting on your knees or thighs (pages 22–25). Close your eyes and start to watch your regular breathing pattern. Notice how it deepens and becomes slower as you relax.

❷ Take your breath to your heart region. As you inhale, feel the area pulsate with positive energy. As you exhale, feel peace filling your heart. Imagine your heart is expanding and glowing with light. Continue breathing in this way until the feeling of peace can no longer be contained by your heart.

❸ As you inhale and exhale, let the feeling of peace spill over into every part of your body. Let it drop into your abdomen and pelvis, seep into your toes and fingers, and fill up from your throat to reach the crown of your head.

❹ As you exhale, imagine the feeling of peace as an energy force, flowing out from the third eye situated between your eyebrows and into the room. Saturate the whole of the room and everyone in it with this sensation. Take an inhalation and feel the love, compassion, and peace still strong within your heart area. On the next exhalation, send the healing energy outside the walls of the room to your immediate environs.

❺ As you inhale, think about areas of conflict and the millions of people worldwide who need your thoughts. As you exhale, visualize the positive energy of peace radiating out and reaching those who need it. When you feel ready to finish, sit quietly, contemplating the connection between yourself and the world and seeing how physical boundaries are able to dissolve.

## chant down babylon

The mantra of peace "Om shanti, shanti, shanti" is said to work first within your own body to nurture calmness and contentment, detox the body's subtle energy channels, and alleviate physical and mental stress. Try chanting it aloud, under your breath, or silently in times of stress or when you want to spread a little peace and goodwill. Try coordinating it with your breathing, uttering "Om" on the in breath and "shanti, shanti, shanti" on the exhalation. Alternatively, use the Hebrew mantra "Shalom," meaning "peace," or just say the word "peace" itself.

"When the TV news makes me feel powerless, I meditate and hope I'm making a difference."

Tracy, garden designer

"The kingdom of God is here, within you."

**Luke 17:21**

# prayerful meditation

- **Giving thanks**
- **Just listening**
- **Praying without ceasing**
- **Chanting the divine name**

The distinctions between meditation and prayer are very fine, and devotional meditation has a role in most of the world's religious traditions in stilling the mind and drawing the devout toward the presence of God. This might be through silence, contemplation of holy words, the repetition of a mantra or sacred formulae, or the passing of beads through the fingers. Unlike in prayers of petition, when you actively ask for help and advice and expend effort searching for beautiful words with which to honor God, during meditation you just are, ready to listen and be filled with an awareness of the divine aspect of everything.

# giving thanks

One of the easiest ways to incorporate devotional meditation into your spiritual life is simply to give thanks daily. Say grace at meals, feel gratitude for those you love on waking and retiring to bed, lift your wineglass to the heavens before drinking, and celebrate the changing seasons with the new growth of spring and the fruits of harvest. When you do this, you interrupt the ceaseless flow of work deadlines, family responsibilities, and all those other demands that numb the senses and brain, punctuating the day with awareness of what's really important.

❶ Sit or kneel comfortably upright (pages 22–25). Adopt your regular prayer position with your hands, if desired. Close your eyes and focus within, watching the flow of breath move in and out of your body evenly.

❷ When you feel calm and centered, start to count your blessings. Think first about your body. Start at your toes and work up, examining each muscle and bone and seeing how most of your body is free from illness and pain. Give thanks for this.

❸ Recall all the beings who make your life enjoyable: family members and friends, coworkers, and people you don't know, those who brew your coffee and bake the bread you eat. Think about people who have enriched your life in the past: relatives, teachers, caregivers, doctors, friends, and lovers. Say "Thank you."

❹ Think about the activities that make your life a pleasure: reading and the gym, gardening and sports, listening to music and dancing. Express gratitude to everyone who makes these things accessible to you. Before opening your eyes, vow to bear these things in mind throughout the day to lift your mood whenever you feel sad, angry, or self-pitying.

## using set words

When repeating a prayer you know well, work slowly, dwelling on each phrase. Examine the words as you pass over them, understanding the resonances afresh and thinking about who they are addressed to. If something seems particularly full of resonance for you today, stop and ponder it. Just be; you may feel you are in the presence of God. Take out phrases that might be useful in everyday life and let them become your mantra for the day. When the familiar becomes unfamiliar in this way, you can glean fresh meaning and awareness each time you pray.

"The same stream of life
That runs through my veins
Night and day
Runs through the world
and dances in rhythmic measures."

**Rabindranath Tagore**

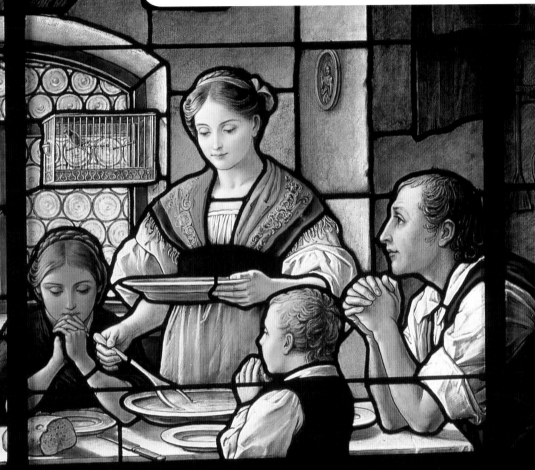

"My kids have really taken to saying grace—
they fight over whose turn it is."

Maria, mother

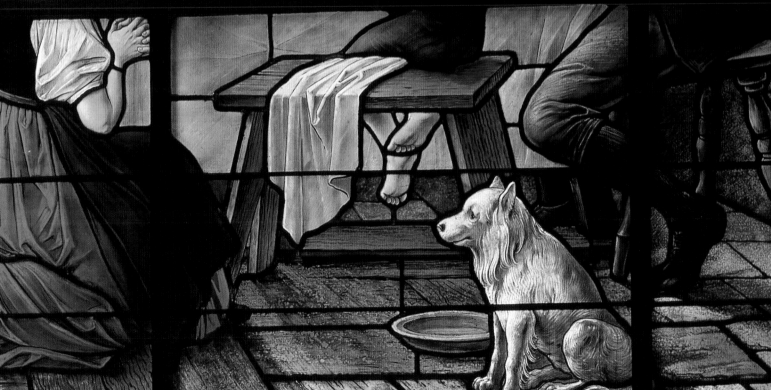

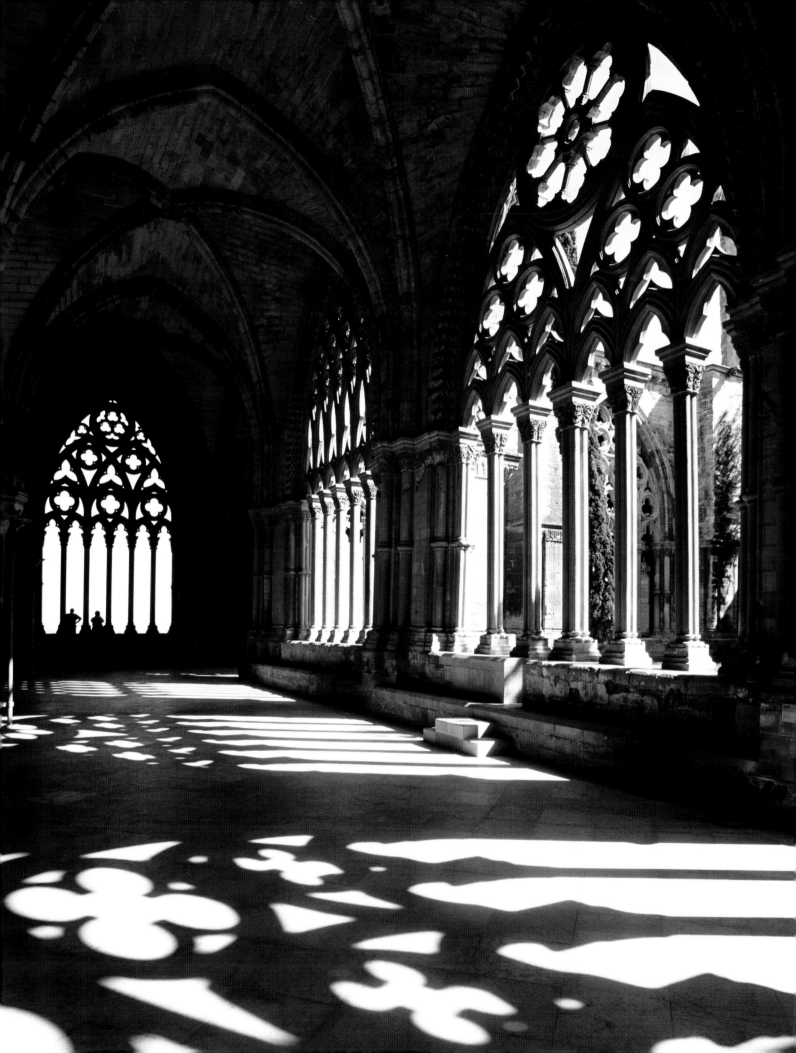

# just listening

Simply being silent, still, and open to God, leaving behind your thoughts, preconceptions, and set prayers, can be enormously fruitful. In this form of meditation, you escape from people and conventions and become aware only of yourself and of God. You are stripped bare, ready to be remade. This may not be your main form of prayer; see it instead as a form of retreat you reserve for a special day of the week. This meditation works particularly well in a spiritual setting, such as a church or a circle of stones.

❶ In your place of worship or at home, adopt your usual prayer position, closing your eyes. Take your attention to your breathing, following the flow of breath in and out, using this to block out other thoughts.

❷ When you feel calm and ready, become aware of yourself. Feel the inner you, stripped of worldly thoughts and preconceptions. It may help to imagine yourself as you were at birth. Touch the spirit of holiness that resides within each of us.

❸ Retain this self-knowledge. Then turn your mind to God. If this seems beyond you, you might get there by focusing on a subject such as love or forgiveness. As you become more receptive, allow God to draw closer to you. Just listen.

❹ Every time other thoughts encroach, come back to your awareness of yourself and of God; eventually the two thoughts may merge as one.

## contemplating holy words

If you feel drawn to sacred texts, use them in your contemplation. Apposite thoughts can be found as you leaf through books such as the Bible or Koran, the Buddhist Sutras or the Bhagavad Gita. Keep some or all of these books in your meditation space for days when you lack inspiration or need some spiritual sustenance and guidance.

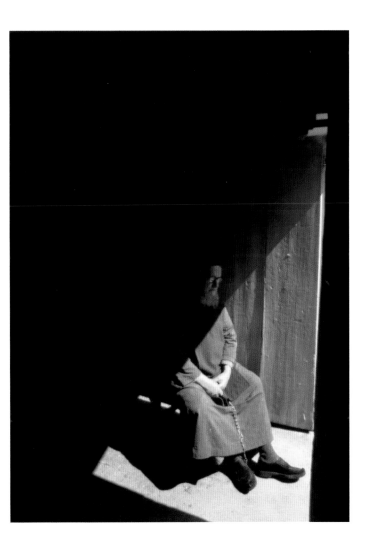

**left:** Constructed in the thirteenth century, the high ceilings and thick stone walls of La Seu Vella in Catalonia keep the noise of the outside world at bay, making it a perfect setting for silent meditation.
**right:** Cistercian monks adopt a simple and largely silent life when they enter a monastery: silence has been described as the mother of prayer.

# praying without ceasing

In many traditions, the aim of prayer is for it to become continual, resonating like an everlasting chord as you go about your daily activities. Across the faiths, one reaches this state by reciting a short prayer over and over until it is fixed in the mind and takes on a life of its own. The Jesus Prayer from the Eastern Orthodox church is one such example that people from many denominations find useful. Repeating its simple words is said to still a wandering mind and quiet a busy brain, fixing head and heart on one point, Jesus Christ. By linking it to your breath, let the prayer invade your whole being, bringing about a profound sense of fullness and inner peace.

❶ Sit or kneel comfortably upright (pages 22–25), adopting your regular prayer position with your hands. Close your eyes and turn inside to watch your breathing. Let this center you in the here and now.

❷ On an in breath, repeat the words silently or in your mind: "Jesus Christ, Son of God"; on the out breath, complete the sentence with the words "have mercy on me." Say the words slowly and with intent. Pause on each one to savor its associations. You may find you want to get to the essence of the meaning by shortening the words, repeating simply "Christ" and "have mercy."

❸ Utter the words on each inhalation and exhalation as your breathing pattern slows and lengthens. Be attentive. When your mind wanders, simply return your focus to the words and their meaning. Work for as long as feels comfortable. You will find that with time and practice, your mind returns to the words effortlessly and involuntarily.

## watching yourself

Stand back occasionally while you pray and catch yourself in the act. See how good it makes your body feel, note how relaxed you are. Allow this knowledge to spur you on.

"I can't get it out of my head. It's so much better than the usual trash that fills my mind."

**Thalia, sales representative**

**right:** Modern architectural designs in churches, such as this stained-glass ceiling, can be used to aid the interior journey with a simple and repeating design that calms the eye and mind.

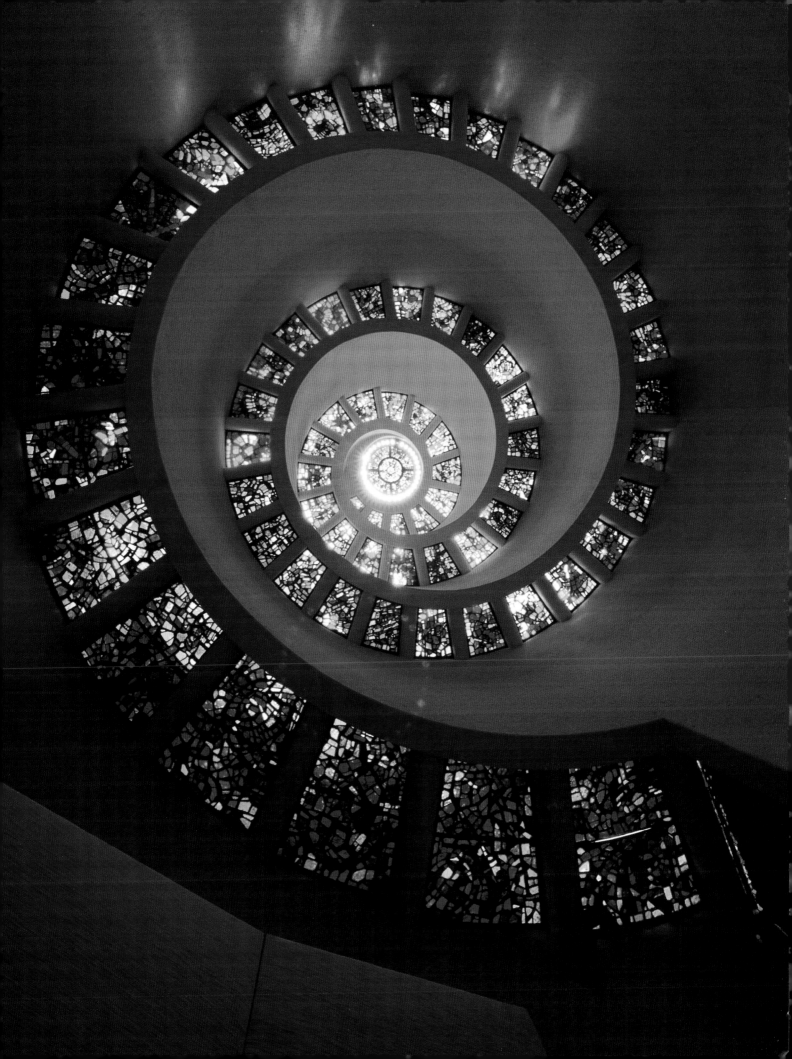

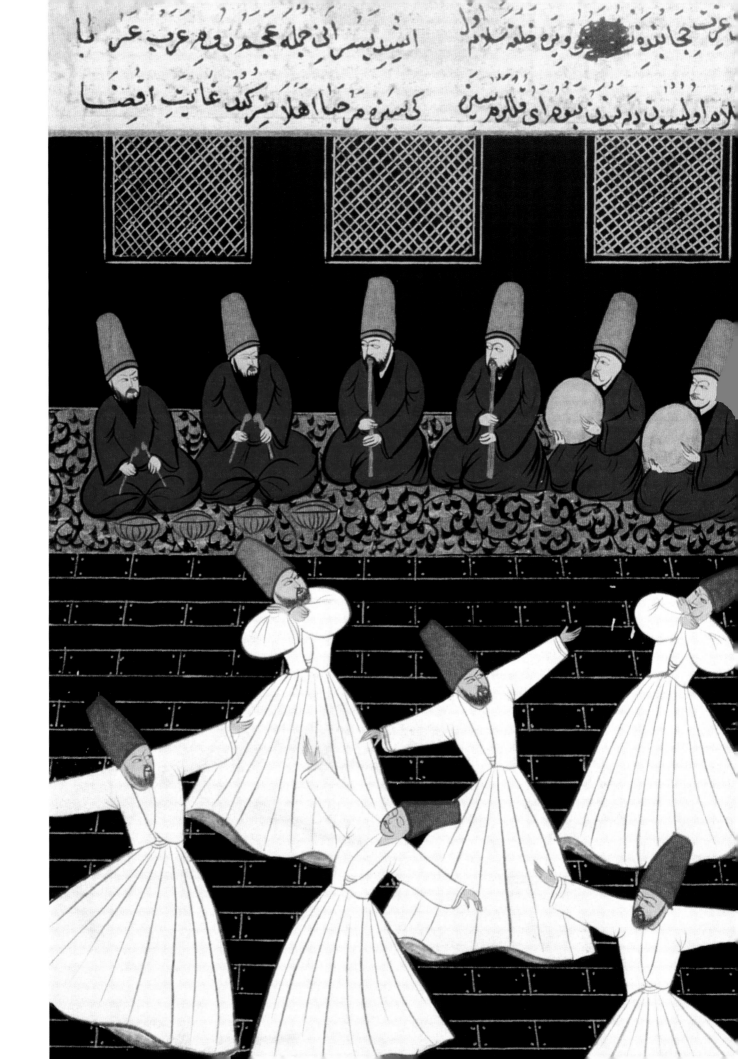

# chanting the divine name

The divine name is thought across the faith traditions to contain at its core all the qualities of the supreme—it is God. It therefore has the ability to evoke in the human mind these very qualities when repeated with faith, and so is at the core of prayerful meditation, such as the bhakti devotion of Krishna worshippers. In many traditions, you seek first to empty yourself, then to imprint on your being the essence of God by repeating over and over the divine name. This meditation is based on one of Christianity's earliest prayers, reintroduced to the canon by the pioneering teacher of Christian meditation, Father John Main. It uses the Aramaic term *Maranantha*, meaning "Come, Lord" in the language Jesus spoke. Feel free to substitute a word that feels right for you.

❶ Sit or kneel comfortably upright (pages 22–25), adopting your regular prayer position with your hands. Close your eyes. Turn inside to watch your breath, noting how, with time, it becomes quiet and deepens.

❷ Clear your mind of thoughts and sensations. Each time something distracts you, come back to awareness of your long, slow breaths in and out.

❸ Start to say the word in your mind on an exhalation, dwelling on each of the four syllables: Ma-ra-nan-tha. Let the in breath come naturally and say the word again. As you repeat the phrase over and over, link it to your breath and anchor your attention to the sounds, feeling them resonate within you. Imagine the words taking root in your heart.

❹ Whenever thoughts arise or you are distracted by your body, simply return to the words and fix your attention on the turning syllables. Work for up to thirty minutes; it is considered most effective to build up a daily practice with this word on waking and before sleep.

## remembering god

People following the mystical Sufi path within Islam work to merge with God using a form of meditative prayer known as *dhikr*, or "remembrance." Phrases or words are repeated over and over, often linked with the flow of breaths in and out and the beating of the heart so that there is no awareness of the ego; the flame of the self is extinguished before God. Some Sufis work with the ninety-nine names of God, others with the fundamental declaration of faith, "La ilaha illallah" ("There is no god but God") or the phrase "Yaa malik" ("O king of kings"). You might prefer to use the word "God," "Lord," or "Beloved."

## calm amid the flow

You don't have to be a Muslim to interrupt what you're doing five times a day and recenter yourself. At those points in the day when there's a natural hiatus or change—on waking and before sleep, at lunchtime, midafternoon, and after work—stop what you're doing, quiet your body and mind, and look inside. Watch your breath move in and out for a few seconds, check your mood, and say a prayer. If you catch yourself doing something you don't like, stop it. This need only take a few seconds, but keeps you in touch with what's important and keeps stress from building up.

**left:** As this sixteenth-century miniature painting shows, dancing dervishes employ a variation on the repetition of chanting: meditative dancing. Ceaseless whirling empties the ego as the spiritual seeker strives to be reunited with the source of creation.

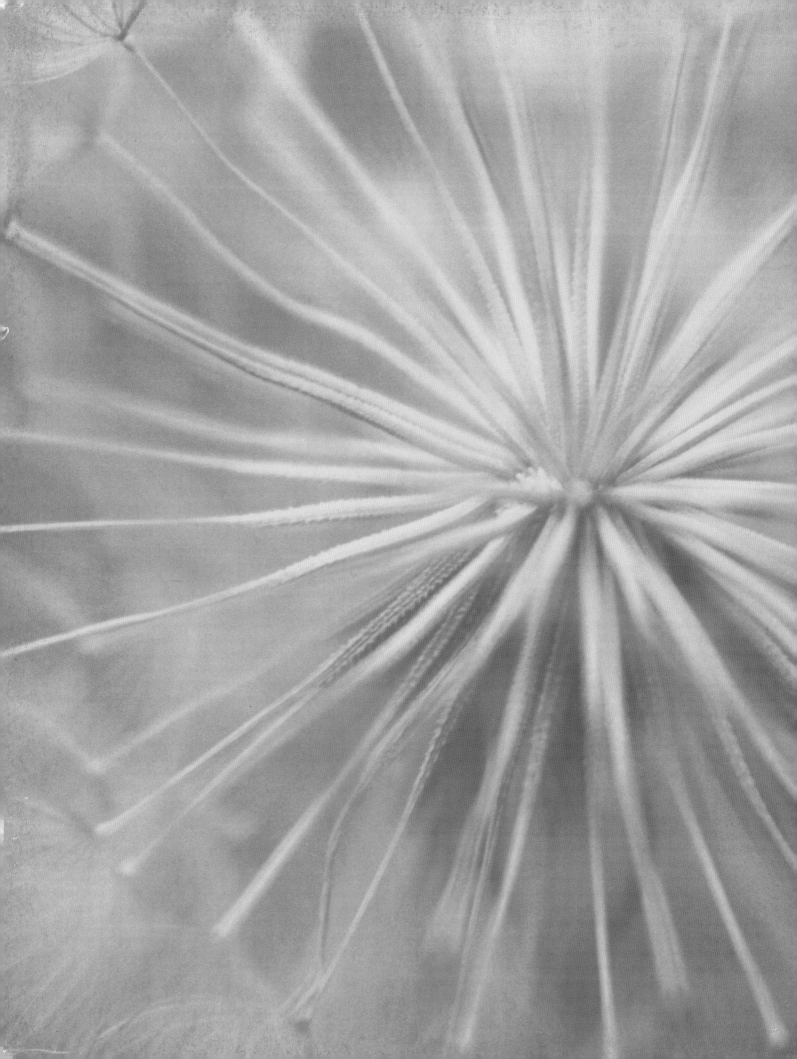

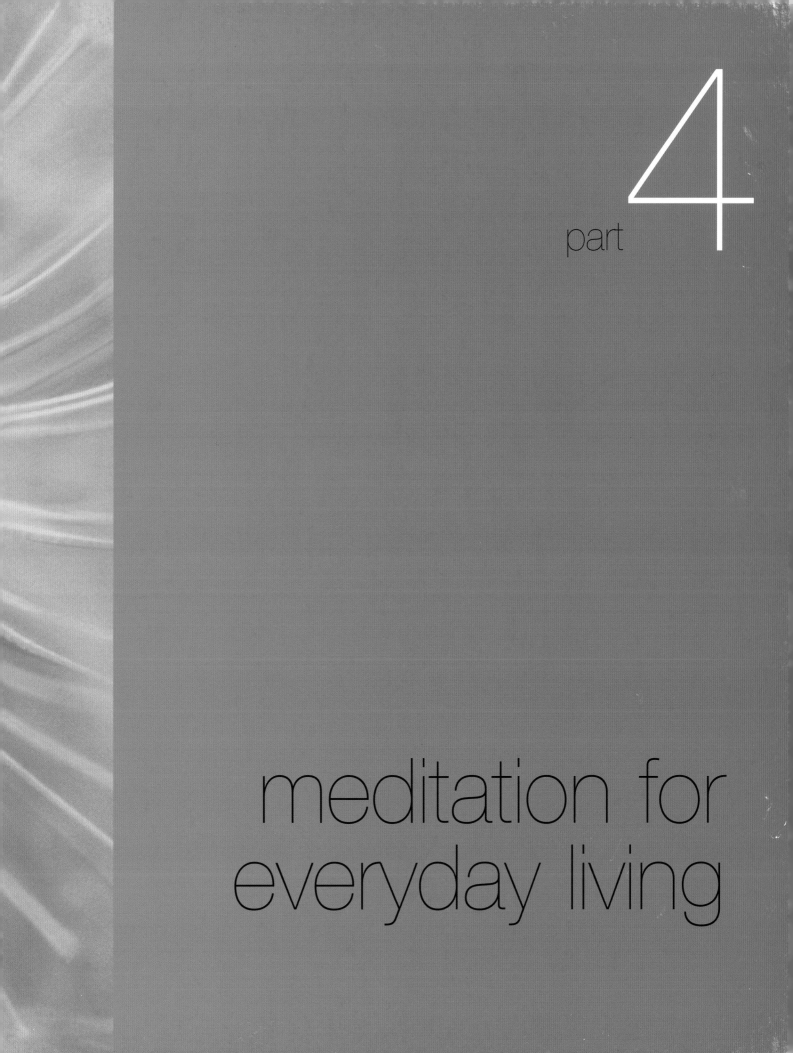

part 4

meditation for
everyday living

# meditation throughout the day

"I'm too busy to meditate!" we all cry. Yes, we lead full lives, but in twenty-four hours you can spare five minutes or so. As the spiritual writer Ram Dass says, even when you're busy, you make time to change the baby's diaper or file your tax return because these tasks need to be done. Meditation should be as urgent a necessity. Plan for it, setting aside a meditation space in your home and daily calendar until it becomes habitual. Soon your meditation space will be inside you. Here are some ideas to help you weave meditation exercises from this book into your day.

## in the morning

Start and finish the day by attuning yourself, even if just by chanting the word "love" a couple of times or showering mindfully. Try building these activities into your prebreakfast schedule (get up a little earlier to make time).

- **Give thanks** for another day, then vow to yourself to use the next twenty-four hours only for good acts. Decide on three things you want to achieve by the end of the day and three things to avoid.

- **Ground your body** by aligning your posture first thing in the day; every subsequent action becomes easier (page 76).

- **Salute the sun** by jump-starting your body with some solar energy (pages 82–85).

- **Use music meditation** by listening to a morning raga while you make breakfast, or play something that inspires you to move, so your heart and lungs are working and your spirit is soaring (pages 72–73).

## at lunchtime

Only one in three workers takes a lunch hour. Make sure you grab a break in the middle of the day to get away from your desk, eat, and inhale some fresh air. This raises your energy levels and ability to concentrate during the afternoon.

- **Cook consciously** and prepare a packed lunch with loving attention so that it tastes better (page 107).

- **Taste meditation** is good for the digestion, too (page 68).

- **Meditate in nature** by taking a nature walk to help free up your creativity and provide solutions to insoluble problems (pages 74–75).

## meditation to go

Don't feel you have to meditate sitting in a set place. Free yourself up by meditating while you sit on a bus, on the treadmill at the gym, or when stuck in traffic. Your day gets happier—and so do the people you interact with.

- **Listen** and let the sounds around you draw you into a heightened state of awareness (page 71).

- **Walk** with awareness—the simple act of walking can free your mind (pages 92–95).

- **Keep in touch** with yourself and the energy of the universe by using so-ham meditation (page 114). Tie in a mantra with your breath as you go about your daily activities.

"I'm overwhelmed by how much happiness I can get from myself every day now that I meditate. I used to rely on others all the time."

**Dave, carpenter**

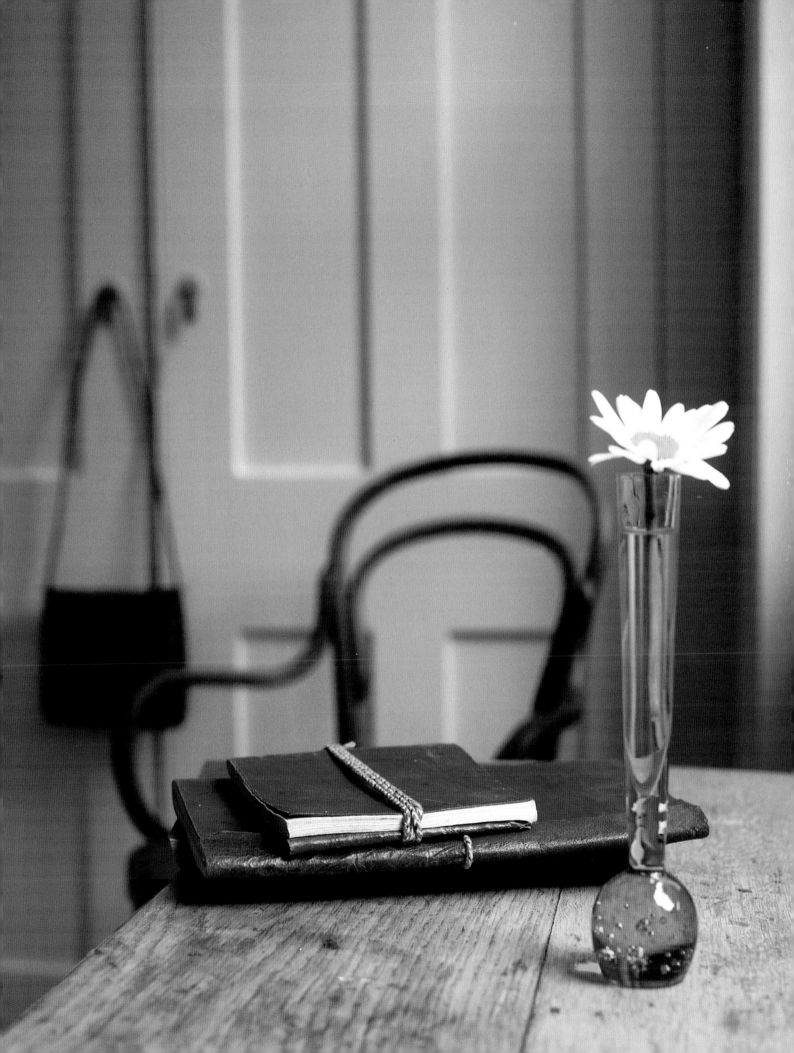

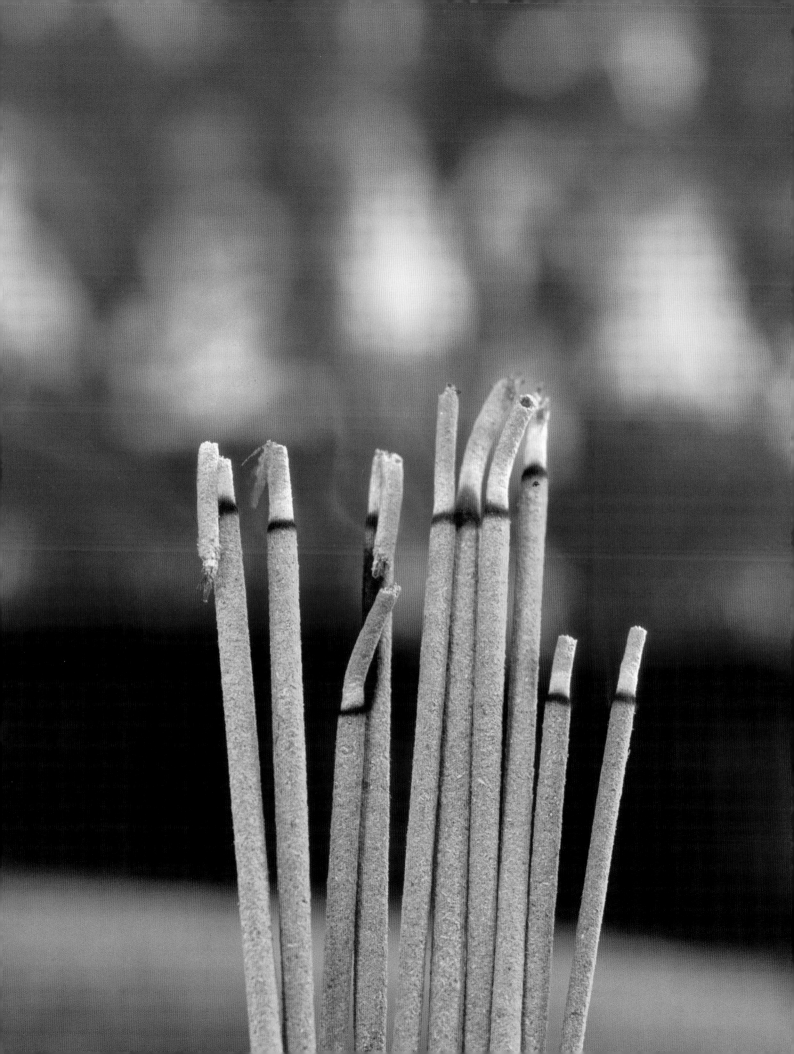

## five-minute break

Every so often during the day, take a few minutes off to step away from what you're doing and watch how your mind is working. Use this time to refocus, find your emotional center of gravity, and check whether you are working toward the goals you set on waking.

● **Just sit** and come into the present and watch your thoughts and emotions as if projected on a big screen (pages 40–41).

● **Draw within** at different points in the day by spending five minutes appreciating every sensation and impression, then let them go (pages 78–79).

● **Count pebbles** or other small objects; use them to tie you to the present and block out the ceaseless babble of thoughts (page 42).

## after work

You might set yourself a mantra to recite as you come through the door each evening to remind yourself of your priorities: "Relax," perhaps, "Just be," or "This is me." Stick a note on the door to prompt you. Review your day soon after you return home, watching it with disinterest like a movie, discerning where you could have made changes for the better. Then let it all go and come into the present.

● **Barefoot walking** is especially effective if you've been standing on your feet for long hours (page 76).

● **Meditation with a candle** can help burn off stress (pages 46–47).

● **Incense meditation** can change the vibes in your living space (page 67).

## before bed

End the day as you began it, by reminding yourself of the stillness at your core and resolving to do better tomorrow.

● **Sit still** and experience the perfect wind-down for the mind and body (pages 40–41).

● **Scan your chakra energy centers** (pages 120–21) by releasing muscular tension in the yoga Corpse Pose, then letting go of tension here too.

● **Count your assets** and check out how you fared on the karma front today; ask yourself whether you missed out on chances to further the goals you set on waking (page 42).

● **Use music meditation** as you prepare for bed by choosing some soothing sounds or a traditional Indian evening raga to lull mind and body into relaxation (pages 72–73).

● **Practice the corpse pose** with the music meditation or when you are in bed (pages 28–29).

● **Say a prayer** at the end of each day (pages 157–61).

# meditation at work

Bringing meditation into your work life promotes efficiency by focusing your brain in the here and now and keeping you aware of your priorities. Research shows that workers who meditate get better results and report increased job satisfaction. Meditation also improves your relationships with colleagues: the techniques keep you poised and cheerful and help you counter unhelpful emotions such as intransigence and anger.

## in a meeting

Don't fall asleep or get agitated; use these quick fixes to boost your brainpower and keep your body alert.

- **Say a silent mantra** under your breath; chant a word that promotes efficiency and clear-sightedness, such as "Focus" or "Energy," or one of the chakra seed sounds (pages 120–21).

- **Breathe deeply** when you can't control your reactions; control your breathing and it will do the job for you (page 113).

- **Cross your legs** under the table. Alter the cross of your legs and arms to keep your brain alert (pages 22–23).

## at your desk

Stick affirmations and instructions to your computer monitor, reminding yourself to breathe and just relax, or try the following ideas.

- **Wake your brain** with a jolt by pondering the impossible using a Zen koan (page 56).

- **Pin up a mandala** above your desk (change it every week) and spend five minutes each morning or afternoon following its geometric intricacies to rest and revive your brain (pages 52–53).

- **Bring nature indoors** and place a bunch of seasonal flowers, twigs, or growing bulbs on your desk to remind yourself of the bigger picture (page 75).

## coffee break

Make the perfect cup of coffee; let mindful awareness and the scent of measuring out and tamping down the ground beans clear your head. Relish every sip, allowing it to erase from your brain all other sensations and thoughts.

- **Relax your body** by tensing and releasing every muscle for a quick but complete relaxation (pages 28–29).

- **Just breathe** and follow the basic breathing advice, especially if your shoulders are scrunched and your stomach is knotted with tension (pages 30–31).

- **Meditate with nature** by going outside at some point during the day to commune with the sun, wind, and rain (pages 74–75).

- **Energize your breathing** with the alternate-nostril breathing technique, working through the active right nostril (page 115).

## to resolve problems

Whenever you feel situations spiraling out of control, step back, close your eyes, and watch the day and your relationships panning out. If you don't like what you see, redirect your actions and thoughts with these techniques.

- **Be yourself again** by stopping and centering yourself to remind yourself of who you want to be (pages 134–35).

- **Just smile** and let this exercise rid you of negativity, and watch how it lightens every relationship (page 138).

- **Develop compassion** and extend loving kindness, which fosters your ability to empathize and connect with others (pages 148–49).

- **Share** a practical exercise with a willing colleague (pages 144–45).

## when things get to be too much

If everyone's screaming at you, the phones are ringing, and there's no escape, try these techniques to let the stress flow over you.

- **Use yoga sense withdrawal** to regroup your mental faculties and slow your heart rate (pages 78–79).

- **Count your breaths** in order to calm your body and get on top of a situation (page 112).

- **Think before you speak** by stopping, diffusing your anger, and only then reacting (page 141).

- **Give yourself compassion** with a treat (page 147).

- **Expel mental toxins** when you feel mentally polluted by zapping your inner enemies (page 140).

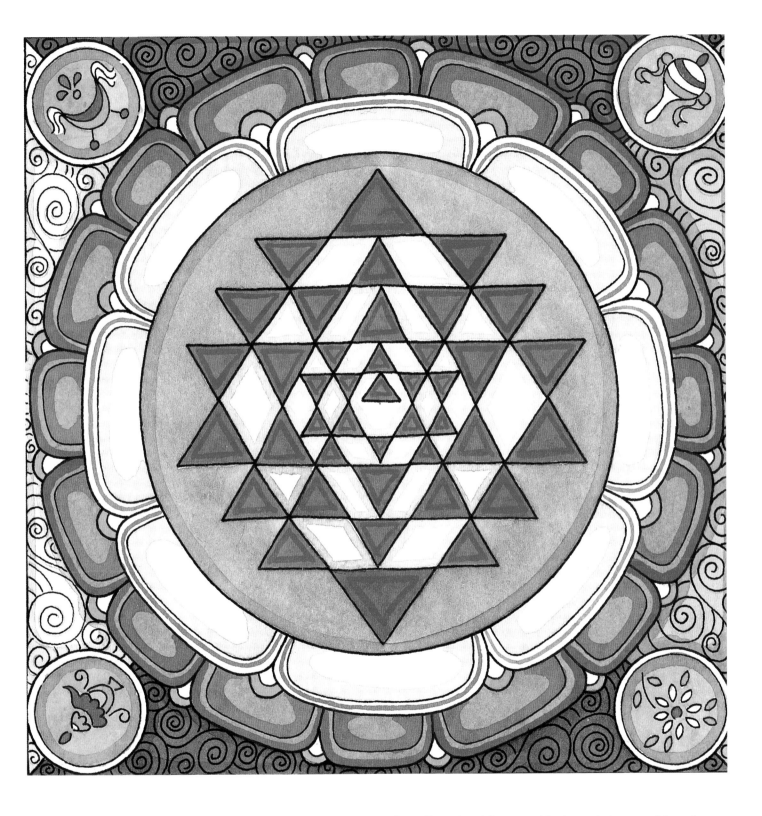

**above:** By contemplating a mandala at your desk you can join up those moments in which you lose yourself in the present and rediscover your innate sense of peace, calm, and tolerance.

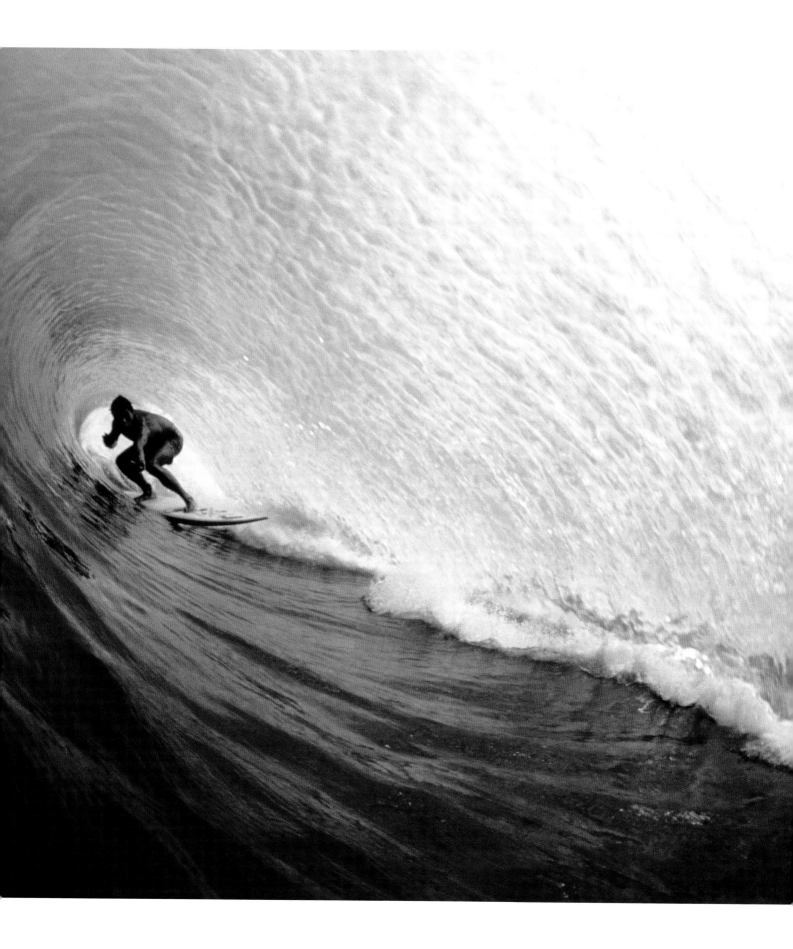

# meditation for sports

Have you ever experienced the sensation of being fully aware as you competed in a sport or during a workout in the gym? You feel like a surfer who has caught the perfect wave: everything is in harmony—your body, your focus, your balance, the environment. Take inspiration from these brief glimpses; meditation can bring you such insight and equilibrium to enhance your performance, banish your fears, and build the patience, enthusiasm, and technique that will help you be the best you can possibly be.

## warming up

Before you warm up muscles and joints, engage your brain and start to channel your vital energy.

- **Align your posture** by sitting upright, with your lower body firmly rooted to the ground. This allows you to focus on stretching the spine out of the pelvis, extending it from its base to the crown of your head (pages 22–23).

- **Start to breathe** with even and deep breaths; every movement becomes easier and actions start to flow (page 113).

- **Use the qi gong exercises** to ground yourself and focus your energies (pages 90–91).

- **Set goals** for what you want to achieve and fix it in your mind by meditating before a game or workout (pages 34–35).

- **Still the mind** and erase other thoughts as you prepare for the game (pages 34–35).

## team-building

By meditating, you can switch off your individual take on issues such as competition and winning and see how it transforms team spirit.

- **Forge partnerships** by practicing yoga as a team in order to get to know each other (page 144).

- **Breathe with a partner** and link yourselves through the breath (page 144).

- **Develop empathy** by watching out for the other members of your team (pages 148–49)

- **Zap self-importance** by making sure everyone works together. This can aid in widening your viewpoint (page 137).

## as you play

Practice these techniques before your game so they come to mind quickly when you need them.

- **Be mindful** of every movement of the arms and legs. Allow the repetitive nature of your actions to draw you away from distraction and hone your game. Adapt this technique to match your specific sport (page 92).

- **Adopt a mantra** by imprinting on your head and heart a word that expresses what you want to achieve, such as "Solid," "Power," "Fearless," or "Smooth." The more often you chant it, the more readily the word sticks (page 119).

- **Stop analyzing** your technique, for it gets better when you suspend conscious thought and just intuit; learn to do this by connecting with your breath while you play (page 113).

- **Learn patience** and make your game more effective by retaining control (page 138).

- **Channel anger** by using negative reactions to spur you on (page 141).

## for injury and loss of form

On those days when nothing goes right and you end up injured or not performing well, think positive with these potential solutions.

- **Visualize pain relief** by thinking away physical injury and mental blocks (page 126).

- **Take a shower** and visualize your problems being washed away with the water (page 100).

- **Expand your mind** to see beyond current issues; watch them evaporate (page 137).

# meditation on the move

Once you are accustomed to meditation, it will come in useful anywhere: standing on a crowded train, waiting in line, sitting at the airport. Let calmness and equanimity replace frustration and physical tension, creating for yourself a portable oasis of relaxation and well-being. And when you can work with eyes open, no one need know what you're up to.

## for endless journeys

Meditation works particularly well in the hermetically sealed space of a car or among strangers on a train or bus. Turn off your cell phone and the radio, resist the urge to shout at red lights and bad drivers, and just be.

- **Meditate silently** by taking the time to be still in silence. Listen to the clamor of the world beyond you and feel the peace of silence (pages 40–41).

- **Counter frustration** by closing your eyes and focusing on the third eye to expand your patience (pages 60–61).

- **Count beads** using a rosary, mala, or worry beads to occupy restless fingers (pages 44–45).

- **Pray** and be open, letting the divine spirit touch you (page 158).

- **Contemplate uplifting words** by picking a quote from a holy text, such as the Bible or Koran, and let your mind unravel it during your journey (page 157).

- **Stretch out** your limbs when you arrive, using a yoga sequence (pages 82–85).

## through the window

Use the time you spend commuting or traveling as an aid to your inner journey.

- **See afresh** and pay attention to the visual world passing by, letting it expand your awareness (pages 60–61).

- **Stop reading** and focus your senses in the present with a listening meditation (page 70).

- **Make a pilgrimage** by using a different route, one that passes by a place that makes you feel good: a spa or temple, a beach or forest (page 92).

## on the street

As you walk along a busy street or hurry to an appointment, use time between destinations to diffuse tension and reset your mind and emotions back to neutral.

- **Walk with mindfulness** by refocusing your priorities and refreshing your brain (page 92).

- **Connect with passersby** as you walk along the street, expanding your empathy for the vast mass of humanity you will never meet (page 147).

- **Stop and be still,** then compare your inner stillness with the frenzy of life around you (pages 40–41).

## on vacation

Vacations can bring stress, as families and friends spend more than the normal amount of time together, and everyday irritants packed in your baggage seem to magnify in unfamiliar surroundings. These ideas may help you escape.

- **Practice yoga with a partner** in order to relax and diffuse tension (page 144).

- **Go on a retreat** every year, spending a day or so alone to rediscover your focus. Spend the time in walking and sitting meditation and eating mindfully (pages 92–95, 40–41, and 68).

- **Enjoy simple pleasures** with a break from everyday demands by taking up a mindful hobby, such as calligraphy or playing an instrument, allowing the careful attention to draw you into a meditative state (pages 99 and 72).

- **Lose yourself** in the beauty of everyday tasks to find rest and renewal (pages 103 and 107).

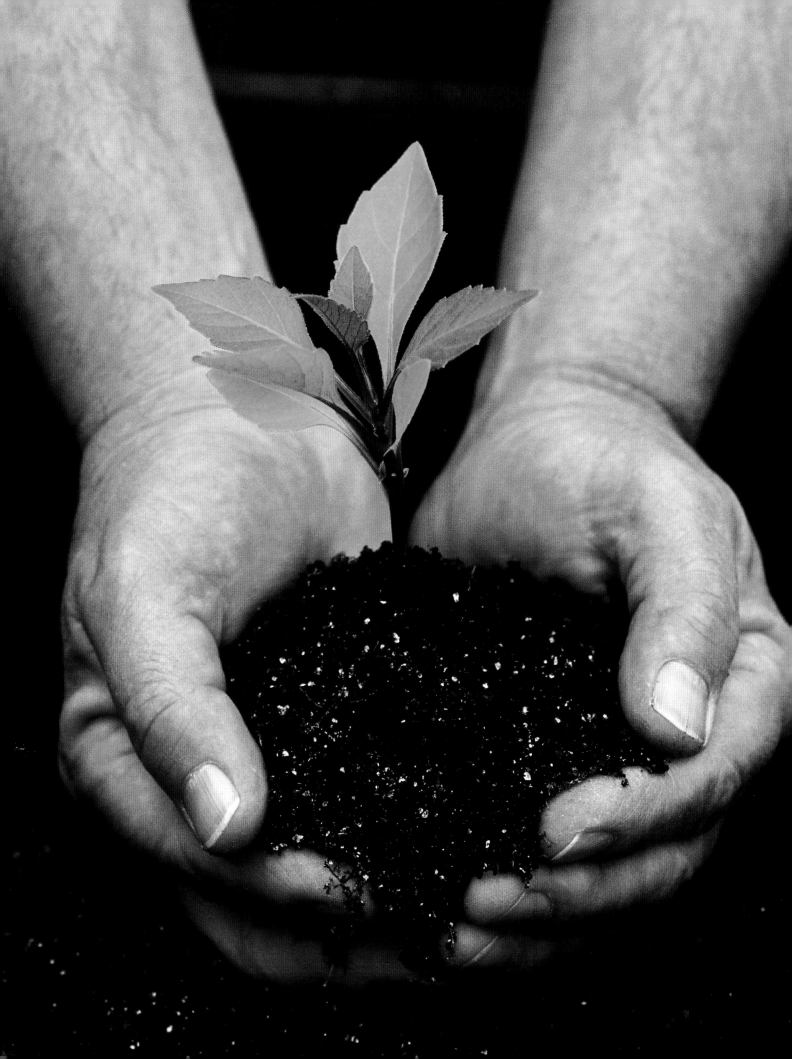

# meditation to bust stress

Most people are attracted to meditation in a search for inner peace, craving a technique that promises total relief from the mental and physical tension that builds up as a result of everyday stress. Meditation is, of course, much more than this once you start practicing, but here are some techniques for the stressed newcomer. Find the resources within to start healing yourself and prevent the many consequences of physical and mental stress, from headaches, back pain, and high blood pressure to unfulfilling relationships.

## unlocking a tense body

For those who think meditation is for hippies, let physical activities start your stress-reduction program.

- **Use progressive muscle relaxation** to let it all go (pages 28–29).

- **Spin off held-in tension** by using whirling meditation (page 88).

- **Stretch your body** by moving and breathing with a flowing yoga sequence (pages 82–85).

## freeing the mind

Wipe out everything other than awareness of the present by focusing on your senses.

- **Use smell meditation** to focus on ambient scents when you feel stressed; draw away from the machinations of the mind (page 64).

- **Practice sensual touch** to ease away stress and tension with a partner by forgetting about everything but the body (page 63).

- **Garden with mindfulness** in order to ground nervous energy with digging, pruning, and mowing, which can clear your mind (page 96).

## sluicing away troubles

When worries are so well rooted that you can't be distracted from them, let very physical actions soothe and cleanse you.

- **Clean consciously** and build up a sweat with vigorous mopping and vacuuming, imagining the sweat carrying away mental and emotional baggage (page 104).

- **Take an antistress shower** to complete the stress-busting treatment. Simply rinse away your troubles (page 100).

## resetting your default

Change the way you deal with stress by getting to understand yourself a little better. In analyzing what causes you stress, you take the first step toward combating it.

- **Forgive yourself** and get rid of guilt (page 140).

- **Find yourself** by figuring out who you are and starting again from a position of power (pages 134–35).

- **Step outside the box** to widen your horizons and the life choices you make (page 137).

- **Appreciate what you have** and just be thankful (page 154).

- **Start smiling** more often; understand that with self-confidence you can change things (page 138).

- **Ask for peace** for yourself first (page 151).

- **Halt the day** so you can monitor your state of mind at regular intervals during the day (page 161).

# meditation for times of crisis

When everything's going wrong or I feel overwhelmed with anger, frustration, or sadness, I tell myself to remember the people to whom this book is dedicated. Haroon died at thirty-four, just as his music career was taking off. Sophie died in her early twenties, weeks after giving birth. This shakes me out of self-pity and reminds me what's important. You will have your own examples to draw from. At other times, these ideas may help you learn to be more at ease with unpleasant emotions.

## facing illness

Meditation helps you understand that nothing is permanent. Just as the days pass, so will pain and the symptoms of ill health.

● **Use healing meditation** to while away time spent in bed and put yourself in a more optimistic frame of mind; self-help visualization can help boost the immune system (pages 126 and 128–29).

● **Think about yourself** and ponder how illness has affected your sense of self, which encourages you to change things you don't like (pages 134–35).

● **Lie in the Corpse Pose** to relax and leave behind the heaviness of the body; sense a lightness as your spirit is freed (pages 28–29).

● **Give thanks** for small things, and thank the illness for giving you the chance to appreciate them (page 154).

● **Try distance healing** even if you're a skeptic; research suggests it can work (pages 128–29).

● **Seek divine help** when faced with illness; Muslims commonly recite the prayer "Yaa Latif," or "O Most Gentle One" (page 161).

## disaster and war

World news keeps us on edge. When you feel helpless in the face of it, reach out to the world with prayer, faith, and wishes for peace. Then back it up with practical action.

● **Meditate for peace** with friends (page 151).

● **Use a rosary meditation** to gain solace through the counting of beads or the contemplation with a rosary of mysteries such as Christ's crucifixion and resurrection (pages 44–45).

● **Give and take** by using tonglen to connect with people you'll never meet (page 147).

● **Harness your fear** and redirect the energy you expend in worrying by using it to create good (page 140).

## accepting grief

Watch yourself in meditation and take strength from your body solidly rooted on the floor or chair and your mind in the present, where nothing can invade it.

● **Just sit** still and silent; although it is hard, it is the only thing to do (pages 40–41).

● **Release everything** by using the Corpse Pose to switch off your body and mind; intuit the essential you that remains untouched by experience (pages 28–29).

● **Gain solace from prayer** in order to empty yourself and allow divine awareness to suffuse you (pages 157–58).

● **Clear out clutter** when your grief is tied up with possessions (page 103).

● **Use your suffering to help others** and offer some relief, even if it may seem unreasonable right now (pages 147 and 149).

## thinking about death

Buddhists say we should all think about death every day to sharpen our awareness and sense of purpose.

● **Imagine your molecular structure** constantly changing; death is just another change as cells merge with the earth and the air. Contemplate this everlasting cycle of change and reabsorption as you meditate (page 35).

● **Divest your sense of self** from your body, mind, and emotions and find your essence (pages 134–35).

● **Free yourself from the senses** to escape from your sensual straitjacket (pages 78–79).

● **Stop the breath** by working to retain it at the top of the inhalation, keeping the lungs empty at the end of the exhalation; appreciate the calm of a state beyond breathing (page 113).

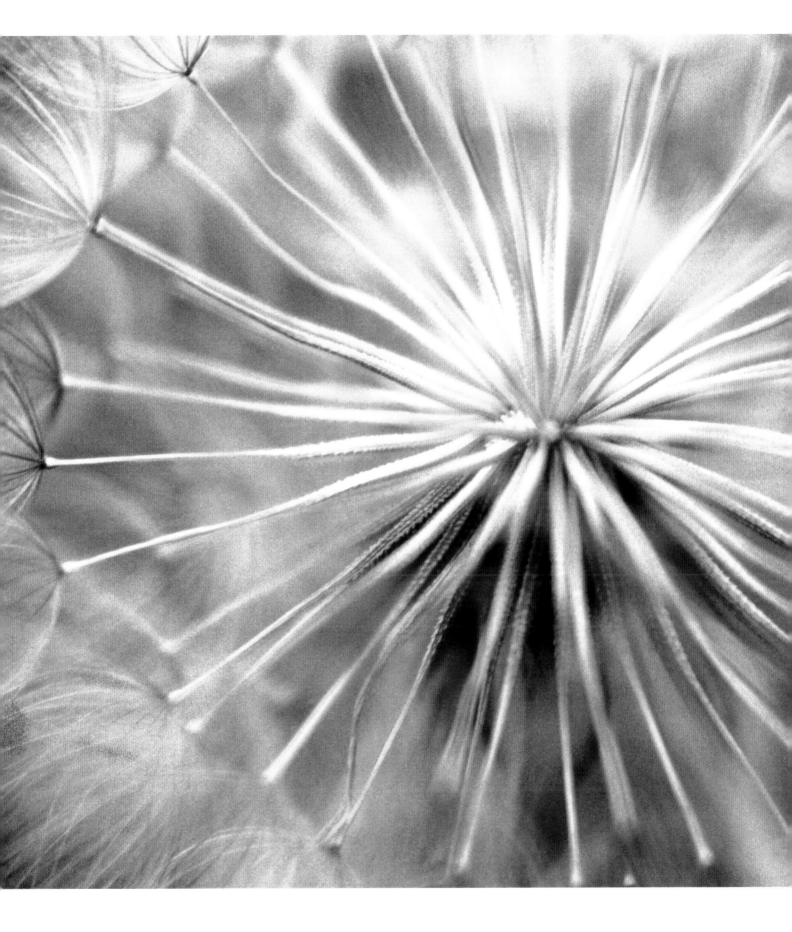

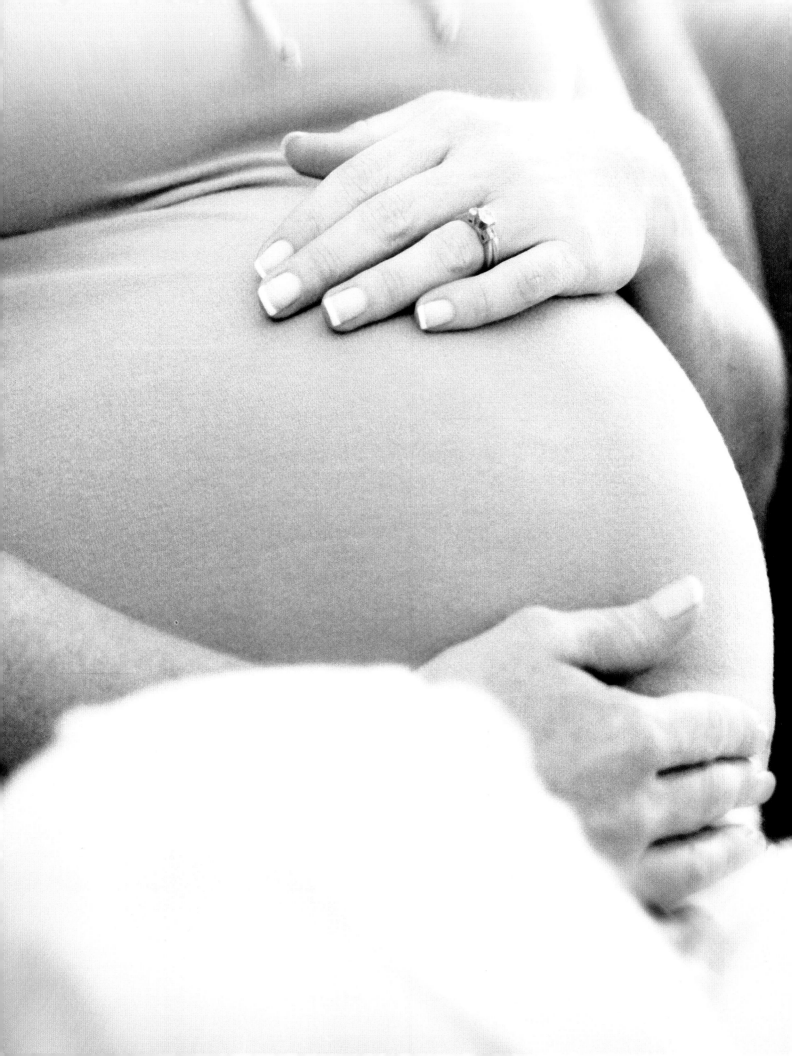

# meditation for mothers

Pregnancy and childbirth should be the most natural and instinctive of states to relax into, and yet many women find this is a time of life that's confusing, tense, and disturbs their sense of who they are and where they're going. These everyday meditation ideas may help you adjust and give up tension.

## during pregnancy

When you meditate, you may find your baby kicks more, enjoying the relaxation flooding through the body. Practice the humming technique throughout your pregnancy so that it is second nature by the time labor starts.

● **Accept your changing shape.** This can be hard for women who work out and watch their weight; find out who the real you is (pages 134–35).

● **Sit and breathe.** Place your hands over your abdomen: as you exhale, cradle your baby by drawing your abdominal muscles back; as you inhale, feel your abdomen rise and imagine love flowing in to cushion you and your baby (pages 30–31).

● **Relax forward.** Sit in the Thunderbolt Pose, then open your knees to each side and relax forward onto a pile of cushions; either meditate here or ask your partner to give you a relaxing back rub, focusing on the lower back and pelvis (page 25).

● **Hum the exhalation.** Sitting comfortably upright with legs crossed, breathe in; hum out the exhalation, making the sound louder as you gain confidence. Feel it vibrate throughout your body. Let the in breath come naturally, then repeat the hum, working for up to five minutes (page 113).

● **Clear the clutter.** Work that nesting instinct (pages 102–103).

## preparing for birth

This is one of the few times in life when you have no choice but to exist fully in the present. Practicing meditation prepares you to ride the waves of pain in labor, going with their opening action.

● **Deepen the breath.** Lengthening the out breath and sounding it out got me through three drug-free deliveries (page 113).

● **Link breaths with a partner.** When you lose sense of everything, this can keep you focused on the task (page 144).

## postnatal period

This can be a terrifying time—breast-feeding in particular seems a particularly frustrating and impossible task at first, and requires reserves of stubbornness to keep going for the hours the baby demands. Meditation keeps you in touch with your core and affords you the confidence to go with your instinct.

● **Use breast-feeding meditation.** When the baby latches on, breathe out your tension and inhale relaxation, particularly into your shoulders and neck; imagine the milk as a copious fountain or a never-ending thread of gold being spun out (pages 30–31).

● **Give up control.** It helps to stop worrying about how things should be done and to erase your own priorities from the picture for a while with forgiveness techniques (page 140).

● **See beyond present difficulties.** If the early weeks seem to drag on forever, try to gain a sense of perspective with spaciousness meditation (pages 136–37).

● **Link breaths with your baby.** When your baby is asleep on you, use this technique, matching four to five of the baby's breaths to one of your own (page 144).

● **Make time for yourself.** Try to find ten minutes a week to be on your own, just sitting (pages 40–41).

● **Get active.** If in the early weeks you get stuck on the sofa, put the baby in the stroller and take a mindful walk or jog in the park to raise your spirits (page 92).

# meditation for children

Children respond well to meditation. Meditation techniques are being introduced in schools across the U.S. and Europe to calm students and boost concentration before class. Teachers report that children take part with enthusiasm and show increased self-esteem and a reduction in bad behavior. If your children don't want to join in, don't force the issue; you may find that if you introduce the technique and then drop it, they'll pester you to try it again.

## for preschoolers

Parents spend much of their time with children crying, "Hang on a minute" while trying to multitask. When meditating with children, don't do it halfheartedly as you prepare dinner—really tune in with them and watch how they respond with every part of the body.

- **Smell meditation:** Try this technique with two- and three-year-olds (page 64).

- **Nature meditation:** When out in the park, point out the uniqueness of the seasons, then take home leaves to print with, sand to make collages, and rocks to put in a pond or bowl (pages 74–75).

- **Breath meditation:** Get a small group of kids together and ask them, one by one, to curl up in a ball on the floor. Have them take turns placing their hands on each others' backs to feel the flow of breath in and out, asking them to imagine a balloon inflating and deflating in their tummies; follow with some games (pages 30–31).

- **Sound meditation:** Use this before a group singing session (page 71).

- **Inner smile:** Young children find this amusing; teach it with a sense of fun (page 138).

- **Just listening:** Take them into a church or temple and just sit and listen (page 157).

## for schoolchildren

At the start of a classroom session, children from the age of five and up can be encouraged to close their eyes, bring their attention into the room, think about their still bodies, and watch their breath.

- **Throwing and catching:** A good way to start focusing; ask children to take every part of their attention to a ball while throwing and catching; talk about techniques such as disconnecting from emotions and letting thoughts pass (pages 34–35).

- **Touch meditation:** Work with children's sense of touch; this is good when done in a group (page 63).

- **Light visualization:** Children find this fun—if you can get them to lie down quietly (page 130).

- **Nature walks:** Take a weekly walk or hike and use the time to look at the signs of the seasons (pages 74–75).

- **Music meditation:** Put on a piece of music and ask children to listen or use their bodies to express the sound (pages 72–73).

- **Barefoot walking:** Children find this easier than adults (page 76).

- **Partner yoga:** Get children to cooperate and learn about sharing and trust (page 146).

- **Clearing clutter:** Clean the room together, using the time to bond and discuss the past, present, and future (page 103).

## for teenagers

If children get into the habit when they are young, it sticks, and meditation can be a valuable way to deal with the stress of exams, broken hearts, and physical changes.

- **Qi gong:** Useful for grounding energy before starting to skate or surf (pages 90–91).

- **Sun Salutation:** Introduce this to teenagers and hope it stays with them for life (pages 82–85).

- **Calligraphy:** Apply the principles here to art projects (page 99).

- **Breath meditation:** Teach the negativity exhalation technique to help them cope with anger and frustration (page 113).

- **Getting to know yourself:** This can be beneficial amid the intense changes of puberty (pages 134–35).

- **Pain-relief visualization:** Girls find this helpful to offset menstrual pain (page 126).

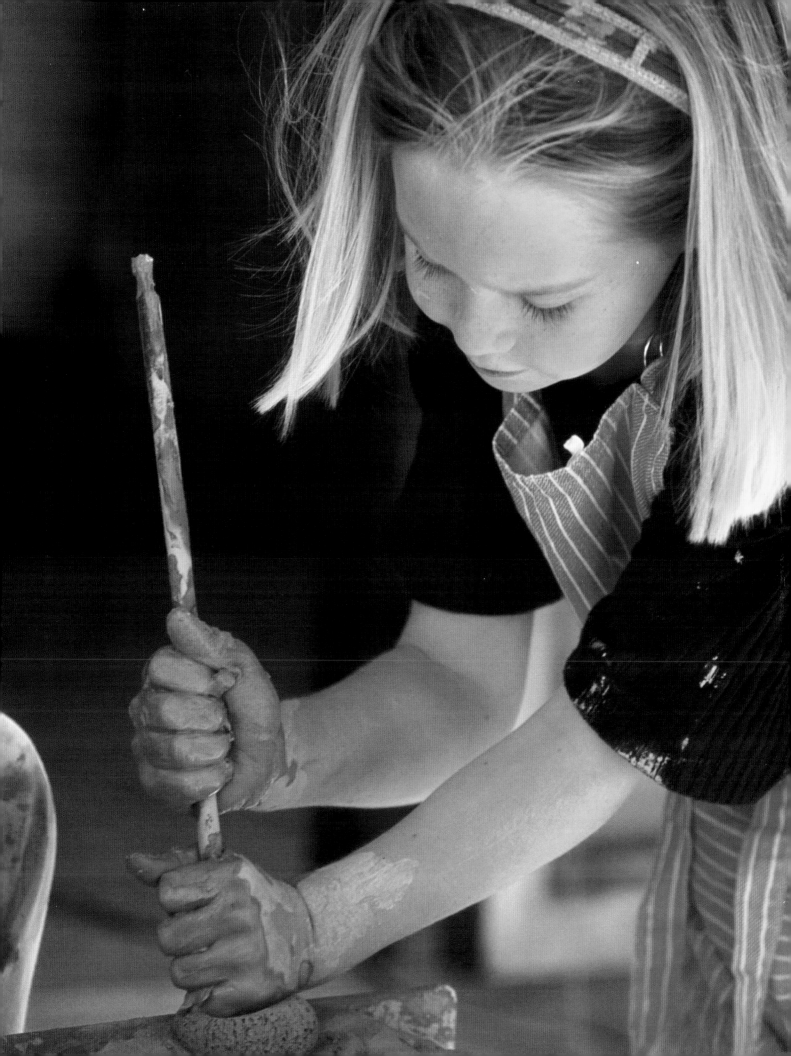

# the tradition of meditation

What's so powerful about meditation is that you use techniques that have worked for people throughout the world for thousands of years. Contemplation, mindfulness, and prayer are bound up with the teaching of the world's great religions. In all, you aim to transcend your individual consciousness and merge in a state of pure awareness with the life energy of the universe.

## meditation in Buddhism

More than 2,500 years ago, Siddhartha Gautama, the Buddha, methodically set out theory and techniques of meditation still used today. Meditation is central to Buddhism; it forms the path to enlightenment or self-realization, the goal of every Buddhist. Meditation cleanses away mental impurities, balances the mind, and fills the heart with love and compassion, bringing about complete understanding, or nirvana—an interior state of permanent bliss, where one is liberated from suffering. The practitioner sees things as they really are.

Buddhist meditation techniques include sitting and walking, prostrating and chanting, contemplating puzzles or patterns, and bringing mindfulness to the simplest acts, such as cooking and eating. In the many forms of meditation, the aim is to become a witness, observing the ever-changing mind and the way thoughts and emotions, sensations and judgments, desires and the cravings of the body affect it. This experience brings self-awareness—of

how you respond to and generate suffering with anger, pride, greed, and selfishness. It also shows that everything in life is ever-changing and so attachment to anything is futile. With this knowledge, one learns to control actions and thoughts, undergoing transformation by cultivating compassion, loving kindness, and serenity to bring about the cessation of suffering within and to extend the same inner peace and love to others.

Forms of Buddhism in different regions of the world teach specific techniques. The Tibetan Vajrayana tradition is known for mantras. The Japanese tradition, Zen, aims to approach every activity in a state of awareness.

Taoism, China's ancient religion, is also founded on living in a state of effortless stillness, forged through learning just to be by sitting in meditation and living according to the Tao, the "truth" and "way." This cultivates an awareness flexible enough to meld to life's twists and turns as they happen.

## "You must learn to be still in the midst of activity and to be vibrantly alive in repose."

Indira Gandhi

## Hinduism and meditation

The Buddha adapted the techniques he taught from Hindu foundations. As in Buddhism, Hindu traditions urge each of us to recognize life as it is—full of hardship, pain, and suffering. Hinduism asserts that each of us is born divine: "Thou art that"—inherently perfect and like God. Our limitations stem from human emotions such as hatred, greed, selfishness, and anger, which result from ignorance of our true state. Meditation and prayer offer one path back to the source. Practice brings glimpses of the divine state and a means to transcend worldly sin and achieve health, peace of mind, and happiness on the way to *moksha*, complete liberation.

Being silent and motionless, practicing yoga, withdrawing from the senses, and chanting divine names or powerful words, or mantras,

often with a mala (prayer beads) are key forms of Hindu meditation. They are reputed to clear the mind, open the energy channels, wipe away sin, divorce the mind from temporal attachments, and lead the practitioner within to a place of stillness and completeness. Here, one experiences a profound understanding of the interconnectedness of all things, and the self comes into union with the divine essence in everything.

In 1957, guru Maharishi Mahesh introduced a secular form of mantra meditation—Transcendental Meditation (TM). It became hugely popular in the West and is said to be practiced by five million people globally. TM has attracted a great deal of scientific research (more than 500 studies in 200 institutions). The technique is always taught face to face.

"It is good to restrain one's mind, uncontrollable, fast moving, and following its own desires as it is. A disciplined mind leads to happiness."

**The Buddha**

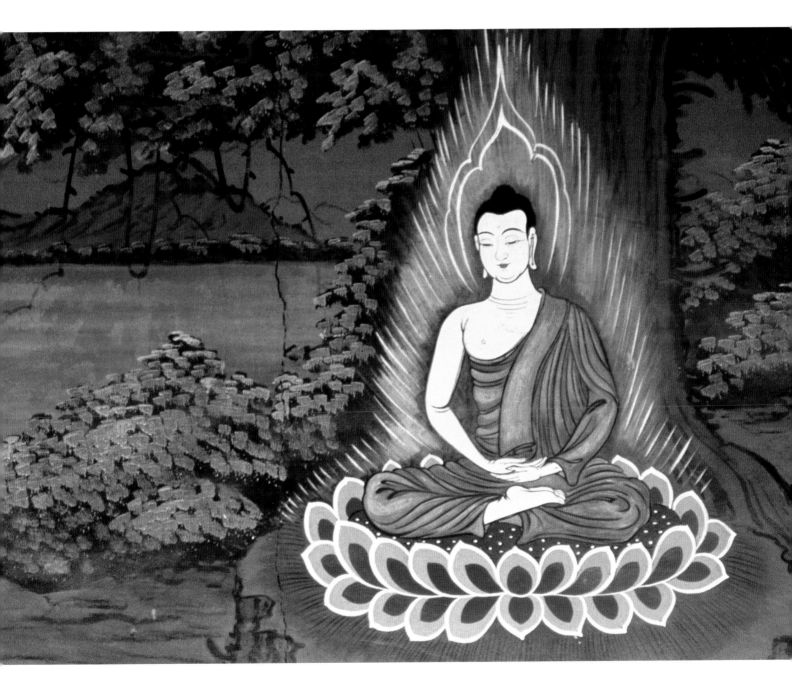

**above:** A painting of The Buddha sitting in meditation; this hangs in the Temple of Yongju, South Korea.

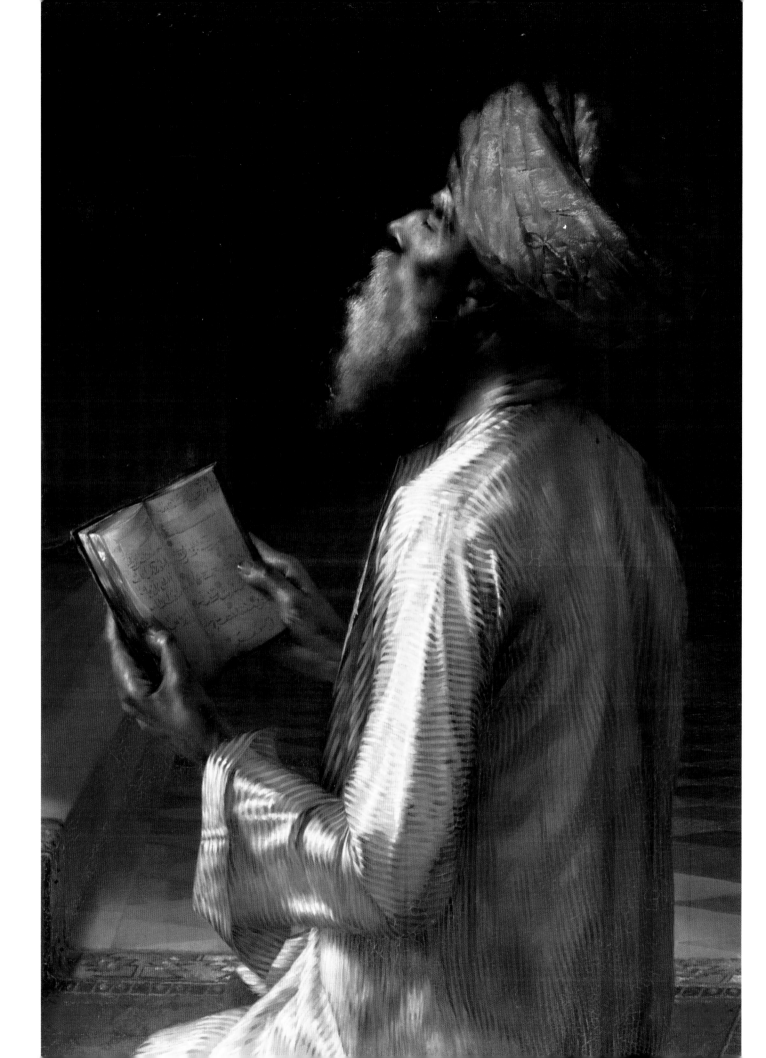

## contemplation in Islam

The five daily prayers of Islam offer a time-out from everyday activities to draw within and let prayerful contemplation bring one into absorption with God (contemplation was likened by the prophet Muhammad to a ladder by which one ascends into God's presence). The Koran explains that in contemplation—*tafakkur*—one reflects on the universe, and the mind, awakened by divine inspiration, develops on a more spiritual plane.

Muslim prayer techniques focus on repetition of the divine name, of sacred formulae that praise God's name, or of verses revealed by God through the prophet Muhammad. Constant utterance while standing, bowing, and prostrating links these words with the breath, the heartbeat, and movement to cleanse body and heart. Every divine attribute is inherent in God's "beautiful names" (there are ninety-nine, all contained in the one name, Allah). These divine names, or qualities, are said to bring the physical world into being. And so becoming absorbed in the repetition of the names draws the chanter into unification with every part of creation.

Seekers on the mystical path in Islam, Sufism, strive through contemplative prayer to lessen the grasp of the ego and imprint on the heart constant remembrance of God, *dhikr*. Repetition of the divine name and meditation on verses from the Koran create a bridge between mankind and creator, and the divine realm becomes all-pervading. One becomes absorbed in God.

"In remembrance of Allah do hearts find rest."

**The Koran 13:28**

## Judaism and meditation

Mindfulness of the divine dimension is omnipresent in Jewish life, and meditation has long provided a spiritual tool to enhance this. Blessings that accompany everyday activities, such as eating or dressing, ignite the divine spark within each earthly act. Reminders of God's commandments sited on the threshold of the home and within the *tefillin* (prayer straps) continually recenter the believer, bringing mind and body into contemplation of God. Through prayer and contemplation, one purifies oneself, enters within to compare oneself with God's commandments, and seeks to rectify mistakes: the word for prayer in Hebrew—*tefilah*—derives from a root meaning "to judge oneself."

A self-work meditation tradition was revived in the mid-nineteenth century in Eastern Europe, in which Polish Hasidic masters taught meditation on portions of the Torah with the aim of perfecting oneself in comparison with biblical figures, better to experience the divine in the everyday world. The tradition enhances mainstream Judaism today, alongside solitary and group meditative practices, including sitting, contemplating the names of God or letters of the divine name, chanting verses, dancing, singing and listening to *niggunim*, or wordless songs. One might contemplate Friday night candle flames, use the Tree of Life personality model, seek healing, or pursue breath techniques that cultivate a state of absence, *eyin*, which is simultaneously everything and nothing.

Increasing numbers of Jews and non-Jews in search of peace of mind, happiness, and spiritual enlightenment are coming to contemplative study of the Kaballah, a body of ancient knowledge thought to contain the spiritual laws that govern the universe and reveal how the divine is intertwined with physical reality.

"And thou shalt love the Lord thy God with all thine heart, and with all thy soul, and with all thy might."

**Deuteronomy 6:5**

**left:** A Mullah at prayer.

## Christian contemplative prayer

The twentieth century saw a reclaiming of the early Christian tradition of silent contemplation espoused by the desert fathers and mothers of the church, but discouraged for centuries. New "centering prayer" movements have sought to make the techniques available not just to monks and nuns, but to the whole congregation.

Key movers in the field include the Cistercian monk Abbot Thomas Keeting and the Benedictine monk Dom John Main, who researched and taught lost Christian meditative techniques to enrich not only those times spent in prayer, but the everyday life and relationships of modern Christians.

Contemplative methods include recitation of a holy, often Christ-centered word, sometimes using a rosary, and ways to cleanse mind and body of unhelpful emotions and ways of thinking. The repetition of sacred words acts to replace thoughts and negative emotions, words, images, and sensations—every part of the ego—with awareness of Christ, of God, and of the Holy Spirit within. The practitioner "rests in God," reclaiming his or her true self: the Bible states that we are made in the image and likeness of God.

Some parts of the Christian fellowship never lost their link with contemplative prayer. Quaker meetings center around shared silent meditation, or "silent waiting." The Iona Community in Scotland devotes time each Sunday evening to a service of quiet prayer in which worshippers sit quietly, turning inside and trying to become more receptive to God.

With the Catholic rosary, the devotee focuses fingers and mind on the recitation of set prayers, including the Lord's Prayer, the Hail Mary, the Apostle's Creed, and doxologies. The repetition of holy words stills the mind and fills the heart. On certain days the believer contemplates with the rosary the Mysteries, defining events in the life of Christ and the Blessed Virgin. In the Eastern Orthodox tradition, the Jesus Prayer (now adopted throughout the church) is imprinted on the mind and heart (it is also known as the Prayer of the Heart) through constant repetition, often with the breath and prostration. One lives the prayer in the pursuit of hesychia, a stilling of the heart that leads to union with God.

"There is nothing so much like God in all the universe as silence."

**Meister Eckhart**

"Then you will know the truth, and the truth will set you free."

**John 8:32**

**right:** A seventeenth-century painting of a votive offering.

Crispino da coldmacio
e sua dona lucia abotirse
alamadona. subito furo
liberati: 1548 —

# resources

## books and cds for beginners

Adamson, Eve, and Budilovsky, Jan. **The Complete Idiot's Guide to Meditation.** New York: Alpha Books, 2003.

Bodhipaksa. **Guided Meditations for Developing Calmness, Awareness, and Love** (CD). Exeter, New Hampshire: Wildmind, 2002.

Fontana, David, and Slack, Ingrid. **Teaching Children to Meditate.** London: Element, 1997.

Hope, Jane. **The Meditation Year.** London: MQ Publications, 2001.

Paramananda. **Change Your Mind: A Practical Guide to Buddhist Meditation.** Birmingham: Windhorse Publications, 1996.

Ram Dass. **Journey of Awakening: A Meditator's Guidebook.** New York: Bantam Books, 1990.

Suzuki, Shunryu. **Zen Mind, Beginner's Mind.** New York: Weatherhill, Inc., 2002.

The Sivananda Yoga Vedanta Centre. **The Sivananda Book of Meditation.** London: Gaia Books, 2003.

## useful web sites

**www.tm.org**
The official U.S. site for Transcendental Meditation, including lists of teachers and courses.

**www.sahajayoga.org**
All about Shri Mataji Nirmala Devi's simple technique for awakening kundalini energy and bringing the physical, mental, emotional, and spiritual into balance. Includes a guided meditation and information on meetings.

**www.shambhala.org**
Resource on Buddhist meditation, with down-to-earth explanations for the beginner, plus guided meditations. A good starting point for further study.

**www.wildmind.org**
An accessible and well-written guide to Buddhist meditation, with audio meditations, online courses, and book links.

**www.dhamma.org**
Highly recommended site teaching the ancient tradition of Vipassana meditation.

**www.zenspace.org**
Step-by-step instructions for zazen, kinhin, and other Zen meditation practices.

**www.wccm.org**
The World Community for Christian Meditation, with a weekly online meditation group.

**www.rebgoldie.com**
Rabbi Goldie Milgram offers an introduction to the tradition of meditation in Judaism, with sample meditations and details of classes.

**www.kabbalah.com**
An introduction and history for the complete beginner, plus course details.

## photo credits

Robert Beer: page 61

Corbis: front cover, pages 11, 12, 16, 21, 33, 34, 41, 48, 49, 57, 58, 65, 66, 73, 77, 78, 80, 89, 93, 97, 101, 104, 110, 122, 124, 127, 128, 136, 139, 142, 145, 146, 149, 150, 156, 157, 159, 160, 170, 173, 178, 181, 183, 184

Getty Images: pages 50, 94

Karen Trist/Lonely Planet Images: page 118

# index